44 Years On The Frontline of Medicine

I0393249

44 Years On The Frontline of Medicine

Dan Andrews MD

Copyright © 2014 by Dan Andrews MD.

Library of Congress Control Number: 2014908292

ISBN:	Hardcover	978-1-4990-1539-3
	Softcover	978-1-4990-1540-9
	eBook	978-1-4990-1538-6

All rights reserved. No part of this book may be reproduced or transmitted in any form or by any means, electronic or mechanical, including photocopying, recording, or by any information storage and retrieval system, without permission in writing from the copyright owner.

Any people depicted in stock imagery provided by Thinkstock are models, and such images are being used for illustrative purposes only.
Certain stock imagery © Thinkstock.

This book was printed in the United States of America.

Rev. date: 06/09/2014

To order additional copies of this book, contact:
Xlibris LLC
1-888-795-4274
www.Xlibris.com
Orders@Xlibris.com
612570

Contents

Introduction

I've wanted to be a doctor for as long as I can remember. My mother claims it started when I was two or three and she had a major surgery. I did vary between wanting to practice medicine and wanting to do medical research but no further than that. My schooling varied quite a lot when I was young, ranging from public schools in small towns to the Agnes Russell Center, which was an experimental school associated with Columbia University in New York where my father got his doctorate in music education. I also spent one year in the school used for teacher training at the small college where my father taught.

The school in New York was very different because they were very liberal. We called the teachers by their first names and would plan each morning what we were going to do that day. I suspect that's part of the reason I can't spell. We never wanted to study spelling.

We did, however, have the resources of the university behind us, so when we wanted to study nutrition, we had lab rats and were supplied with food mixes to our specifications. Because our schedule was tied to the university's and not to the public schools', we would be off when they were in session. One time my friends and I wanted to go to a movie on our day off, but the theater wouldn't let us in because the public schools were in session. We finally found a foreign film theater that would let us in, and they really gave us an education as well.

New York was the first place I really came in contact with hard-core racial prejudice. Even the building we lived in (which was owned by Columbia) had all-black maintenance men and the only black family in the building was in the basement apartment, a fact that meant nothing to me but which they had not failed to notice and which one of their boys commented on.

I also got my first job there carrying a paper route for a couple of blind ladies who owned a news stand on Amsterdam Avenue. I got paid a whole dollar a week for delivering about ten to twelve papers a day. Not much work until the *Sunday Times* showed up. Since my route passed the edge of Spanish Harlem, it was a little bit dangerous (something I made a point of never telling my mother). I was held up three times by kids with knives and was very careful not to carry any money or candy with me. Even though I was always pudgy, I learned to run fast especially when the other guy had a knife.

By the time I got to junior high, I was back in the public schools in our town in eastern Washington. I maintained my keen interest in science and had some problems with it. In the seventh grade, we had a science teacher who simply didn't know his subject so I decided it was my duty to correct him. The man must have been a saint because I would have killed a little snot who acted that way. The science teacher in the eighth grade knew his material but was very strange in other ways, including being a neat freak. He had us keep these huge notebooks, and since my handwriting was as bad then as now, he wanted to flunk me in science. Since I had never missed a question on any exam including bonus questions, I felt this was very unfair. My parents and the principal finally convinced him this was unacceptable and I got my A.

When I got to high school, I started a science club, and since it was my idea, I got to be the first president. Several of my friends and I also organized a debate club, which got us out of class for trips. When I was a junior, I was involved in setting up the junior-senior prom and developed the idea of a fountain in the middle of the gym. We put a couple of washtubs of hot water in the fountain and added dry ice at regular intervals, which resulted in a mist over the dance floor. Unfortunately, it also got the gym floor wet, which didn't make the janitor and principal very happy with me. My interest in medicine never left me, to the point that I signed up for two years of Latin, thinking it would help me later. Not only was it a horrible experience, it wasn't much help either.

I'd always wanted to earn my own money, so in junior high, I had a paper route carrying eighty to eighty-five papers daily, rain or snow. The system was such that the paper took no risk. The carrier had to pay for the papers and collect the money. If someone didn't pay, that was too bad; the paper didn't help. Sometimes you'd have to return to the same house three or four times in order to collect. By the time I turned sixteen, I had a job at a local filling station back when you pumped the gas and washed the windshield and checked the oil. I got a whole dollar an hour, and in the three to four years I worked there, I never got a raise even though I eventually was responsible for hiring and firing the night shift.

By the time I was a senior in high school, I started going to the college where my dad taught. We had what was called advanced placement courses, but at that time, it meant we went to the campus and took honors courses with the college students. I managed to finish a year of math and a year and a quarter of English by the time I graduated from high school. Because I knew I would be going to medical school (arrogant, huh?), I decided to get through college as quickly as possible and live at home, since we lived in that town, so as to save as much money as possible. As soon as I graduated from high school, I went on to a full load at the college in summer school. I majored in biology and had minors in math and chemistry. I also joined the college debate squad and soon was elected captain. After the first year our coach quit and we had to find a facility advisor. I found a professor who said he didn't know anything about debate but was willing to sponsor us, so I became the coach for that year. I also gave up my job at the filling station in favor of a job as the biology department's laboratory assistant.

College went fairly smoothly as I went year round in hopes of finishing in two years, but by my last summer, I decided to take the summer off and work. I also had taken the Med CAT test (I never even knew there was such a thing until the head of biology asked if I had signed up but I must have done OK). Subsequently, I was given the chance to interview at all three medical schools I had applied to. The medical school I finally chose had interviews that were the roughest, and I learned later they were designed that way to see how you reacted to pressure. There were eight applicants in each interview group, and we had four interviews, each lasting about twenty minutes with twenty minutes between each interview. Less than half the total applicants were even asked to interview. My first interview was with the chief of medicine (very famous but known to the house staff as Dr. Malignant). I found his office, and since it was Saturday, there was no one at the secretary's desk, so I timidly knocked on the door of the inner office. He was sitting in a high-backed chair facing the window and away from the door. He apparently had my transcript and spun around with his finger pointing at me and said, "Andrews, why do you want to go into medicine instead of music where you belong?" (I had taken several music courses in college.) The interview went downhill from there. I learned at the end that half the interview group had left without completing the whole process.

Fortunately, I was accepted at all three schools where I'd applied, but my ultimate choice was considered as good as any school in the country, so I decided to go there.

That winter I took a light schedule because I was close to having enough credits to graduate anyway. The summer before med school, I helped my dad build a summer cabin at a lake north of Spokane, and having already received my book list, I started studying my books for the fall. I made arrangements to live in the Phi Chi House (a medical fraternity). This was very cheap lodging and included meals. Come fall I thought I was ready to go and was very enthused. Boy, did I get that knocked out of me in a hurry.

This book is largely made up of memories. I didn't keep notes or charts, so if memory is a little self-serving, please keep in mind that we all remember the good things better than the bad and see ourselves in the best light possible. I have tried to be honest, but I'm only human too. Many of the people discussed are still alive, and I have avoided the names of people and places, although anyone who really wanted to could, I'm sure, figure most of them out. If I've wronged someone, it wasn't intentional, and I will apologize ahead of time. I'm reasonably sure no one will be able to figure out who the patients are and their privacy will be protected. I've changed some of the circumstances and locations to prevent any loss of privacy.

Medical School

The first day of med school we were assembled to hear the dean discuss what was expected of us. We were to wear black slacks and white shirts. He then looked hard at one of the guys from Phi Chi who had arrived with a full beard and said, "We have always been proud of our student's *clean-cut appearance*." Needless to say, the beard was gone by that afternoon. We were shown around the school, including the gross anatomy lab where there were twenty complete bodies for the eighty students and numerous partially dissected body parts for demonstration. This experience was somewhat of a shock. A couple of people fainted, and even though I had dissected cats, fetal pigs, and various other animals, including searching through the entire contents of a cow's gut to find parasites for the biology department, real people were different, and I got very light-headed for a while.

The courses were arranged so that the first year we studied the normal such as human anatomy, physiology, histology, biochemistry, and normal psychology. The second year would be spent in abnormals such as pathology, abnormal psychology, pharmacology, bacteriology, and so on. We were required to take the full set of classes, which amounted to twenty credits or so of graduate-level classes. Other graduate students were only allowed to take twelve. We also had a small number of electives, which you could add if you wanted more.

After the day of orientation, we jumped right into the fire on the second day. We started with the anatomy lecture. I was feeling pretty good because I'd read the first 100 pages of the book and thought I would be ahead, but the professor opened the lecture by saying he knew we'd all been studying the book so we would be held responsible for the first 150 pages on the exam, but he was going to start his lectures on page 151. I'd been in class only a few minutes and was already 50 pages behind. That was just a taste of what was coming.

We finished our morning classes and were scheduled for gross anatomy lab for the afternoon. In the lab we were assigned to a cadaver—two students on a side. Our first assignment was to skin the chest and get the muscles so they could be seen. This included removing fairly large quantities of yellow fat. When we got done, we went home with the smell of formaldehyde clinging to us like a special medical student perfume.

Dinner that night at the Phi Chi House was a tradition we freshmen weren't aware of until they served us large plates of corned beef with yellow fat clinging to it. Many of the freshmen had to get up and skip dinner while the upper classmen laughed and hooted. That was the only instance of initiation I remember ever happening there, but it was effective and probably was the only incident of skipping a meal in my medical career.

My lab partner was Jan, one of the women in the class and indeed on the other side of our cadaver was Mary, another of the four women in the class. These slots were decided by alphabetical order and we worked together through most of medical school. There were only four women in the class because the state legislature limited the female slots to 5 percent of the class. Their reasoning was twofold: (1) women averaged a 50 percent dropout rate (indeed two of our ladies were gone by the end of the second year), and (2) women tended to get pregnant and drop out of full-time medicine and the legislators wanted physicians who would practice full time. Today about 50 percent of medical students are female and such limitations would be thrown out as unconstitutional. It is still true, however, that many female physicians don't work full time.

Anatomy lab soon became routine to the point students would go there on their lunch hour to catch up and eat with one hand and dissect with the other. We did have some levity because we had in the class a ventriloquist who had studied under Edgar Bergen (he of Charley McCarthy fame) and occasionally would have one of the cadavers say something. We also had one wag who was working at night when he heard the janitor coming and went to an empty table and covered himself with one of the blue plastic tarps we covered the bodies with to keep them from drying out. When the janitor came in to clean, he just sat up. We had to clean the lab after that.

Physiology lab was also of interest. We had to do experiments, some of which involved white rats. After the experiment, we had to "sacrifice" the animal using a small guillotine designed for the purpose. It was fast but we all hated it. One experiment required human blood samples from a finger stick. I volunteered to provide the sample. The instructor suggested we take it from the side of the finger so it wouldn't bother us as we worked. Jan took the lancet and prepped my finger. She then proceeded to rip part of my cuticle off. Naturally I complained about the pain and asked why she did this. She admitted she'd closed her eyes as she poked me. After that we used her blood.

As a group, medical students are an interesting bunch. The guys in our class had varied backgrounds such as an electrical engineer, an optometrist, and a night club performer. The guy in the room next to mine at Phi Chi graduated from Harvard with a degree in English. He had his own drummer all the way. One time he went skiing even though he didn't know how. He told me he took the lift to the top and just pointed his skis straight downhill and screamed at people to get out of the way because he didn't know how to turn. He also hitchhiked home on the freeway across the mountains. Both ways he got picked up by the highway patrol but talked them into taking him where he wanted to go rather than giving him a ticket. He had an old car that had windshield wipers that only went one way. He rigged a string from the wiper to the wing window, and when the wiper went across the windshield, he would pull it back using the string. That car eventually killed him when he got drunk after finals and wouldn't let anybody drive him home. He crossed the centerline on a bridge and hit five cars head on. He was in the ER for several hours before one of the Phi Chi guys recognized him.

We experienced a very high mortality for a group of young men. In addition to my friend above, the class ahead of ours had a student hang himself from a pipe in the locker room during finals. A senior student committed the most hostile suicide I've seen. He had been in a fight with his girlfriend. She left to go to work. He took some strychnine and lay down behind the door. Strychnine works by blocking all the inhibitory circuits in the brain so lying quietly on the floor in a quiet room, he was just fine until the girlfriend came home and opened the door throwing him into terminal convulsions. We lost one guy trying to get home for Thanksgiving. He'd been up all night in OB and then tried to drive home. He apparently fell asleep on the freeway and didn't make it.

As we worked our way through the year, sleep was a precious and rare commodity. I became a heavy coffee drinker to keep going. I was so stressed the whole first two years my pulse never got below a hundred. We tried to have a party one night each weekend, but that was about the total for recreation.

Phi Chi House was a beautiful half-timbered house located on the boat canal from an inland lake to the sea directly across from the medical school. Inside was not so beautiful. My first room was in the basement where we had a chronically backed up and nonworking toilet. We were afraid to try to get it fixed because we suspected it emptied into the boat canal out back, and if the city found out, we'd have major repairs for which we had no money.

My bed was like sleeping in a hammock; it sagged so far. It was somewhat difficult climbing out. Also in the basement was the liquor vault where the house's store of hard liquor was stored. There was a large lock on the door for which only the house manager had the key. One of the largest bottles was a giant vodka bottle, which held mostly lab alcohol and was the basis of the punch we sometimes made for the parties. Those of us in the basement also got to share with some large black rats. The student in the room next to mine woke one night to hear the throw rug next to his bed moving. When he turned on a light, he found it was being dragged by a huge rat.

The house sat next to a city park, which was on a kind of point out into the bay, and beyond that was the city yacht club where there were many boats, some of them million-dollar corporate yachts with million-dollar girls sunning themselves on the decks. We considered that as medical students we were very eligible bachelors, but the security at the club didn't seem to see it that way so all we could do was watch. That sometimes got worse on Sunday afternoons when we had a ton of material to study and the yachts were going through the canal passing just twenty or thirty feet from where we were working. This really made concentration difficult.

One night at 2:00 or 3:00 a.m. when I still had work to do and was falling asleep, I took my small fishing rod out to the boat canal intending to cast a few times and see if that would wake me up. I had seen locals fishing for bass off the bank in the park. On the second cast, I felt a tremendous strike and the line started streaming off my reel. Fortunately I had more line than the canal was wide. I fought the fish for about forty-five minutes, slowly winching him in and then he'd run across the canal again. When he was finally tired I started yelling for help from the guys in the house, and they came out and helped land this monster. It turned out to be a twenty-one-pound King Salmon migrating from the sea. I cleaned the fish and put him in the refrigerator. He eventually made dinner for the whole house. While I was doing that, I discovered some of my housemates, being good physiologists, had the fish's heart in a glass of salt water at the strength of saline and had gotten it to start beating. They kept it going as long as possible. By that time I was wide awake and able to finish my studying, which was what started the whole episode.

There was a tradition of presenting an unknown slide to one of the professors in histology who, it was claimed, couldn't be stumped. This professor wasn't into deodorant so most of us avoided him when possible, but a group of students made up a slide using some ground up chicken's beak and presented it to him on the last day of class. He studied it under the microscope and said in his thick German accent that the only thing he could think of was ground up chicken's beak, thereby keeping his perfect record intact.

Exam time was total panic time the first two years in medical school. The grading was on a curve, but in the anatomy lab final, for example, 100 percent was an A, 99 percent was a B, and if you didn't get at least 97 percent, you failed. Nobody in our class failed but a couple of anatomy grad students did. The stress resulted in a lot of misadventures. One student looked into a microscope in the histology lab and vomited all over the scope when he realized he hadn't seen that slide before. One guy got so stressed he couldn't urinate and had to be taken to the ER to be catheterized. One student disappeared for three days and was finally found after sitting in a downtown all-night theater for three days. He had to drop out for a year but was told he could come back the next year, which he did, but eventually he dropped out altogether. We even had one student admitted for observation for chest pain.

The second semester I ran into my nemesis, neuroanatomy. I did everything I could think of to learn the various tracts in the brain including diagramming them in all planes in colored pencil, but they wouldn't stick. Fortunately the class was called a conjoint class with neurophysiology. By combining the grades, I eked out a "C" in spite of failing the anatomy section. I never wanted to be a neurosurgeon anyway, but it was disappointing that I spent at least twice the time on neuroanatomy as anything else. I guess I don't see in three dimensions very well and that has never changed.

That semester our anatomy professor became ill and had to take a leave. He was replaced by a little Italian professor with a very big ego. Needless to say, the students didn't like him and his attitude didn't help. He was in the habit of coming in before class and drawing the skeletal anatomy of whatever region he was talking about on the blackboard. One day we came in and found the skeleton of a foot drawn on the blackboard but no sign of the professor. One of the students went up front and drew a sixth toe and a corresponding metatarsal on the board. When the professor arrived, he didn't notice and began drawing the muscles and tendons on the foot in colored chalk including the sixth toe. He finally figured out something was going on when the class kept giggling and stood back from the board. He demanded to know who had done it, but he got no response from the class. In those days it was traditional for the other faculty in the department to attend each other's lectures. Even though they'd been sitting there while the superfluous toe was added, they didn't point out the culprit. I don't think they liked this guy either.

The summer after the first year I landed a job as a research assistant in the public health division. I was especially interested in tropical medicine and particularly in parasitology.

I had heard this department had summer programs in that field when you got further along. My job consisted of developing tests to identify the various strains of mycoplasma, which is a specialized form of organism halfway between a virus and a bacterium. My boss was one of the world's experts in the field and also taught a course in virology I took that summer as well.

The lab was an interesting place with all kinds of people working there. The boss had several projects going at once and mostly sat in his office and thought. He was both a chess master and a bridge master and would join the rest of us for a bridge game at lunch. Playing with him as a partner was scary because it was as if he'd seen every hand during the bidding and would make bids you never thought would work out, but they always did.

In addition to the boss there was a professional lab technician who was working with Trachoma virus. She caught an eye infection with that organism and responded readily to antibiotics, which I couldn't understand at the time because antibiotics don't work with viruses. Subsequently it was discovered that this organism was in fact an obligate intracellular bacterium, which today is called *Chlamydia trachoma*. An obligate intracellular organism cannot grow outside another living cell. We no longer even try to culture it but simply diagnose it with a DNA probe. This organism was once the number one cause of blindness in the world and is still a common sexually transmitted disease.

The woman sharing my lab was a graduate student who was studying streptococcus and growing huge quantities of bacteria in twenty-liter bottles to get enough material for the studies she was doing. One day she left early to go to a tennis date, and that afternoon we heard she was in the hospital. She later told me she had a small pimple on her arm and suddenly went into sepsis while playing. The organism was in fact Strep, which was fortunate because it was so easy to treat in those days.

We had one other full-time lab tech I only saw at lunch and I don't remember what she was working on, but she did have great stories about her cats. She and her husband kept exotic cats, including an Ocelot and an Indian Fishing Cat, which was so big it pretty much did what it wanted because even her husband (an able-bodied seaman) couldn't control the animal. One day she told us she was leaving because her husband had fled to Texas. He'd been diagnosed with active TB and, in Washington State, was required to remain in quarantine for at least six months while he was being treated, and he refused to do that. We never saw her again.

We had a grad student who was also a nun, and since she was very willing to discuss religion, we had long discussions while waiting for a culture medium to cook. She was the first nun I had met who didn't wear the habit but only somewhat conservative dress. She had been something of a fast lady when young and had come to religion later in her life, which perhaps gave her a more earthy view but did not make her any less devoted. Since I had had minimal exposure to Catholics, I learned a great deal from her I had never understood.

Another very significant thing happened that summer. One of the men living at Phi Chi was getting married and we were all invited. Two of us didn't know anybody we could take and felt uncomfortable going to the reception alone where there would be dancing. We finally hit on the idea that we'd call one of the women's dorms and see if anybody was interested. Amazingly enough, this worked. The young woman who was coming as my date was teaching in central Washington and had come to the university for the summer to pursue a master's degree in English. We both felt a little uncomfortable going to a wedding as a first date and stayed at the reception only for a while. My friend and I decided to take our dates to a place called the House of Banjos, which was a favorite of the college students. The floor of this place was covered in peanut shells and the only things on the menu were peanuts and beer. There was a stage high above the main floor where a banjo band played, and they had a drummer with many noise makers such as a siren and a weight he kicked off the stage, which pulled a rope attached to the hammer of a fire bell. A special event occurred when you got the waiter's attention, usually with a five-dollar bill in your hand and pointed to your lady. Soon the band would play a fanfare and a spotlight would go on and find your lady. The waiters would surround the woman and stand her on her chair. They would then put a garter on her as high as they dared while everyone hooted and hollered. The girls took it with good spirits probably in part because we'd been filling their glasses every time they looked away. I have no idea how many pitchers of beer we went through.

Sue and I saw each other almost every night that next week, and on Saturday I cooked a steak barbeque for several of the guys and their girls on the patio of Phi Chi House overlooking the boat canal. Apparently I was the only one who knew what different cuts of steak meant, and I really had to work to get theirs tender because they all bought round steaks the cheapest cut. I had bought T-bone. By the end of the evening Sue and I agreed to get engaged. While we'd only known each other for a week we did wait a year to get married, and now, after forty-four years and six kids, we're still together. I guess it worked out.

My second year in med school was another tough one. We embarked on our studies of abnormal such as pathology, pharmacology, bacteriology, and abnormal psychology. In addition, I became the manager of Phi Chi, which saved me $25 a month and required me to control the finances with the cooks and do what I could to improve things in the house. I also was going frequently to see Susan. I began taping the lectures so I could play the tapes when I drove since I couldn't study my notes. It turned out that worked fine going over there, but trying to listen to a lecture in the dark coming back at the end of the weekend nearly got me killed when I found myself falling asleep. So I had to give that up on the way home.

We had two cooks at Phi Chi, both of them older ladies who were on Social Security. In those days, if you were on Social Security, you could only earn $1,500 a year in additional income. We split the job between the ladies and they each worked half time and only during the school year. Each week I would sit down with the "head" cook and we'd plan the menu for the coming week. We tried every way we could to keep costs down. One trick we tried was to switch to dried skim milk because the guys drank a lot of milk and it was getting to be a major expense. Unfortunately the complaints came fast and furious, but we found if we mixed the dried milk half and half with regular, we could stand it.

We had one luxury that consisted of buying a gallon jug of cheap Mountain Red wine on the nights when we had spaghetti. In retrospect, it doesn't seem like much of a luxury, but back then it was a real treat.

My biggest accomplishment that year was getting new beds for the house. We had some money in our account, and I got a couple small donations from Phi Chi alums in the area. I used these to bargain with a hotel supply company and got pretty good beds for the house.

All medical students were broke and there were a number of ways to make extra money. The researchers had figured out that students would do practically anything for $25, which was usually the going rate. The pharmacology department tested new painkillers while I was there. They would give you $25 to put you in a thumbscrew or a metal head band and see how many screws of the tightening mechanism you could stand. They'd then give you a known painkiller, the experimental drug or a placebo and see if you could tolerate more turns of the screw. One of the things discovered was that the placebo worked about 20 percent of the time. The psych department had a famous annual drug party where you were given a psychoactive drug or a placebo and were in a room with many other people and with observers who tracked your responses. Since in those days one of the psychoactive meds used was LSD, it was more than a little dangerous. Fortunately, my parents were able to help me out so I never had to do any of those things.

The most interesting course that year was pathology. In addition to the regular lectures, on Fridays, all the pathologists in the area would participate in the "bucket brigade." This consisted of each of them bring in a specimen or two that they'd had the previous week and lecturing on the disease. One fellow autopsied a pilot from a small plane crash in the southern part of the county. Purportedly he'd been buzzing the airport and failed to pull up in time to clear some trees near the end of the runway. The pathologist had brought in his heart, which had ruptured with the force of the deceleration. You could still smell alcohol when he opened the bucket. The pilot not only was buzzing the airport, but he was buzzed himself.

Another interesting bucket was a surgical specimen of a twenty-five-foot tapeworm taken from the stomach of an elderly lady. This worm was of the type transmitted in beef and not one of the ones from pork. The lady never traveled and bought all her meat at a local chain supermarket. That's probably why most parasitologists eat only well done meat.

A member of the city's health department was brought in as a guest lecturer in preventive medicine and spent a great deal of time discussing a battle they were having with a cheese company who felt that they couldn't make good cheese with pasteurized milk. The cheese was frequently contaminated with Staphylococcus, and they had had several instances of people getting sick and at least two deaths that seemed to relate to their cheese. The company argued that most people could eat their product just fine and disputed the few cases of sickness as having anything to do with their cheese. The health department physician pointed out the people who got sick were all elderly and not in good health. The health department eventually won and I could not tell the difference in the cheese before or after it was pasteurized.

We had one lecturer in immunology who spent a number of lectures discussing his own research into the rabbit's immune system. We, medical students, were disgusted at the time wasted on this subject until we discovered when we took part one of the National Boards that he'd written a large number of the questions in immunology, and you guessed it, they were about the immunology of the rabbit. I bet we were the only students in the country so well prepped on that subject.

Toward the end of the year, we had a course in physical diagnosis, which consisted of learning to use the instruments we would use the rest of our lives, such as the stethoscope, the ophthalmoscope (used to look at the back of the eye), and more mundane things like reflex hammers. In addition, we had to learn how to take a history with all its parts.

After learning these things, we were taken in groups of four with an instructor and given a patient to interview and examine. For the most part the patients were cooperative and even helpful, except one very large man at the Marine Hospital who had uncontrollable hypertension. After taking his history in which he told us he'd never had surgery, we found on his physical that he had healed incisions in both flanks. When we asked him what those were for, he told us they were from an experimental operation, but he didn't know what was done. When our instructor came in, we presented him complete with his unknown experimental surgery. The instructor asked him about the scars, and he said, "I had a bilateral sympathectomy to try to control my blood pressure." We were furious that he made us look like we hadn't asked the right questions. The instructor said he was a professional patient and did that sort of thing to students all the time.

We also began to get a look at some clinical medicine and discover that the transition from animals to human cadavers was no better than the transition from cadavers to live people. We were assigned one morning to watch the anesthesia prep room, and the chief of anesthesia was to demonstrate a spinal anesthetic on a man going for urologic surgery. The patient was elderly and had arthritis in his spine and therefore was difficult to tap. The room we were in was somewhat crowded and warm, and after a couple of attempts, the chief finally hit the spinal fluid and there was some blood running down. Several of us were bending down trying not to faint. One fellow suddenly passed out hitting his head on the tile floor. They had to disconnect the oxygen from the patient and put it on the medical student.

The National Boards come in three exams, and the first is taken at the end of the second year of medical school; the second, after medical school; and the third, after internship (now called first year residency). The exam lasted most of the day and was broken into parts like biochemistry, pathology, anatomy, and histology. The volume of material was huge, and nearly everyone came out feeling they'd failed.

Our school had year-end final exams, which occurred a week after classes ended, and then another few days before the boards. Most of the week after lectures was spent studying with very little sleeping. I remember one night, at three or four in the morning, when we'd all been studying and were getting sleepy, we decided to run around the block to wake up. The neighbors must have loved having fourteen medical students crashing around the block at that hour. We did try to get a full night's sleep the night before the exams. One of the guys had a bottle of Dexedrine he got from his brother who was a physician, and one night I tried one to keep going. I was very tired and loaded with coffee and the result was my heart started racing and skipping beats. I got on my bed and lay still until it wore off because I thought I'd rather die than go to the ER and admit what a stupid thing I'd done.

We thought the exams were tough until we took the boards. Those exams were composed of questions from a select group of professors around the country. We were fortunate that the rabbit immunology professor was among the group writing questions. I don't know how many of the questions came from our school, but I'm sure a number did. Apparently they analyzed the results and threw out the questions that were missed too often as probably poorly worded. Regardless, when you left the exam, you were certain you'd failed, but as far as I know no one did. We did have one fellow who had an eidetic memory (he remembered everything he had ever read), and he scored so high they wouldn't rank him because he was so far above the curve. It was hell competing with him on a grade curve.

The day after the exams, I flew to Michigan to get married. Sue had set everything up, even getting an exemption from a judge for the waiting period because I couldn't be there any sooner. My family was all there, and Sue's extended family was there, which turned out to be about half of Michigan since her father had many brothers and sisters. I was so tired I really don't remember much of the wedding or reception. Afterward, we flew back to Spokane and honeymooned at my parents' lake cabin, which I'd helped build. A week of honeymoon and it was back to the university and the lab job. We lived in a trailer in a park ten miles north of the university, which introduced the added complication of commuting.

I was back in the mycoplasm lab, but now my assignment was to see which atmospheres were best for culture of these organisms. I would remove all the air from the vacuum container the cultures were in and introduce various amounts of oxygen, nitrogen, and carbon dioxide and see how the organisms grew. For some reason that work was never published, and I am still the only person as far as I know that can culture *M. pnumonae* in three or four days.

My boss was very tall and had the facial appearance of Abe Lincoln. He was used as an example of the appearance of Marfan's Syndrome in the genetics class, but apparently he'd never been told, and since he was a PhD and not an MD, he was unaware until one day he mentioned to me he'd been seeing wavering movements in his vision. Marfan's Syndrome has a problem with weak connective tissue, and one of the places it manifests is in the eye with retinal detachment. I had to explain to him what was thought throughout the school about his appearance and sent him urgently to the ophthalmology department.

I took up wine making that summer and bought special cultures of wine yeast at a local beer and wine store. To stretch out my cultures I grew some in media in our lab incubator. Unfortunately the carbon dioxide apparently built up, and when I picked up the flask, the media erupted all over the incubator. Fortunately, my boss wasn't too upset, but the lab smelled like a brewery for a few days and I had a big cleanup job.

The third year of medical school was devoted to the major areas of in-patient study, including medicine, surgery, obstetrics and gynecology (Ob-Gyn), pediatrics, and inpatient psychiatry. I started right out on medicine and was very impressed with my attending who was famous worldwide for developing the drug ampicillin and for developing a method for testing antibiotic resistance. He turned out to be very nice to the students and house staff, even inviting his team and our spouses to dinner at his house.

The interns helped us with our write-ups, which seemed to take forever. The patients were sometimes somewhat hostile when they were really feeling bad and a student showed up to do the third history and physical behind the resident and the intern. We would make the rounds on every patient, and we had to be able to present the case including the lab results if asked. Fortunately the resident and intern did most of this, but at any time the attending physician could ask the student to present the case if he'd worked the patient up. At this time plans for further tests and treatment were decided with the attending, and after rounds we had to remember what was said and write the appropriate orders.

In addition to the daily rounds with the attending and the afternoon rounds with the resident, there were the chief's rounds once a week. Our chief of medicine was very famous and was a principle author of *Harrison's Textbook of Medicine* and internationally known. It was said he'd graduated number one in his class at Harvard and had an eidetic memory. There was usually an intern assigned to present the case and he frequently put lab data on the blackboard in the meeting room. In one particularly difficult case the intern covered all the blackboards with lab and when the professor walked in he just stopped, stared at all the lab, turned to the intern, and said, "Who the hell authorized you to do a total body lab?" Not an auspicious start.

Sometimes the chief would decide to make walking rounds after all the work the intern had done and take everybody out to the ward, select a chart at random, and ask which resident or intern was caring for this patient. He'd then read the chart and ask questions. One time he picked up a chart and read through it and asked who the resident was who was responsible. When the resident admitted he was, the chief looked at him and said, "This workup is not acceptable on my ward. You're fired." That was the end of that young man's residency at the university. He had to go find an opening in a second year residency elsewhere.

One day we were on rounds with another team on medicine when I managed one of my rare coups. They were presenting a girl with right upper quadrant (upper right abdomen) pain, which had occurred a couple times. Mentioned in the history was that she had had a cold before each episode. The gallbladder was unable to concentrate x-ray dye indicating the gallbladder was sick, and they were about to transfer the young lady to the surgical service for gallbladder surgery. The story struck me as strange, and I asked the young lady if her doctor gave her antibiotics when she got a cold (a terrible practice but common) and she said he did. I then stuck my neck out and bet the assembled physicians that she had been taking Ilosone (erythromycin estrolate). When she was asked, the patient took a bottle of this medication out of her purse. I had remembered that this salt of erythromycin sometimes caused gallbladder spasm and pain similar to gallstones and was considered a form of allergic reaction. The attending had never heard of this but was fair enough to ask for an allergy consult before sending her to surgery. I was told the next day that the chief of allergy had had to look the reaction up but put in his consult that the problem was presumptive cholangina (gallbladder pain) and she should just avoid the medication and did not need surgery.

We admitted a young halfback from the football team who had become jaundiced (yellow from blood breakdown products). After a full workup it was found he had had a blood disorder called Familial Spherocytosis, which made his red cells very fragile. Broken red cells are picked up by the spleen and broken down completely. In addition to his inherited disease, he had caught infectious mononucleosis. The two disorders were breaking down his red cells at a very rapid rate, and in order to handle it all the spleen had swollen to the size of a basketball. The liver is also involved in Infectious Mononucleosis, so he couldn't clear the breakdown products and therefore became jaundiced. The spleen lies in the left upper quadrant of the abdomen and is notoriously hard to feel especially for beginners at physical exams. As word went around, the medical students were flocking to examine this athlete to see what a spleen felt like. The residents finally put a sign on the door of his room advising the students not to examine the patient. Because the spleen was so large it was very friable (easily broken), and they were afraid repeated poking might cause it to rupture.

I had one very difficult problem when my former anatomy professor was admitted to my service. I had thought highly of him while in his class and was unhappy to find he had a disease that at that time was almost universally fatal. I was told I still was required to take the history and do the physical, but after that, his care would be managed by the attending and the chief resident only. He was very gracious and probably less bothered by the history and exam than I was. He did soon die of his disease.

We admitted one man who was complaining of severe chest pain radiating into his left arm, which mimicked the pain of a heart attack. He required fairly large doses of IV morphine to keep him comfortable. His EKG did not show changes indicating heart damage, but it was thought to only be a matter of time until it did. We did not have coronary care units in those days, so the patient was in a room on the regular medicine ward with a heart monitor attached. Those old monitors were shaped like a bullet and would be placed on a stand outside the door to the patient's room. We had just decided to get a psychiatry consult because of the constant complaints of pain without any EKG confirmation when the patient signed himself out of the hospital. The next day the cardiologist who had been handling the case told us he was making rounds on his private patients at a private hospital across town when he was called to the ER, and there was our patient with the same complaints. He had taken a cab directly from our hospital to the ER at the other one. It turned out he was a morphine addict and went from hospital to hospital with complaints, which got him morphine at each one. That probably explained why he insisted on smoking the whole time he was with us since the two adictions tend to go together. Not an option in today's hospitals.

We rotated on inpatient psychiatry the third year, and I drew the inpatient unit at the VA Hospital. They had two wards referred to as the open ward and the locked ward. We were each given a key to the locked ward. This was like a huge skeleton key and we joked it could double as a weapon if we were attacked. That was not entirely a joke because a nurse had been attacked just before we got there and had suffered permanent brain damage. The striking thing was that the attack occurred with the least severe patients who worked outside of the ward during the day but came back to the ward the rest of the time. She was checking them out when one fellow punched her, for no apparent reason, knocking her unconscious. The house staff was barely able to save him from being beaten to death by the other patients for hitting their surrogate mother.

We observed group sessions, including AA meetings, and were also assigned individual patients to work up. My first patient was a manic-depressive who was barely controlled with doses of medication that would have stopped a horse. This patient would go for years in a normal state and then go into a manic phase for no apparent reason. He had some sort of hang-up on musical instruments, and his wife would find out he was going manic when she'd come home and find their garage filled to the brim with various instruments. Apparently he'd go to the waterfront and buy every instrument in all the pawnshops in the area. This time after his obligatory instrument shopping trip, he turned up in his psychiatric social worker's office wearing a pair of cowboy six guns. Unfortunately, they were real and loaded. He walked in twirling them, and apparently, the social worker called the cops while hiding under her desk. One of our psych lecturers said if you interview a patient and come away feeling happier than justified, you had just interviewed a manic, and boy was he right. The interview sessions were full of mirth even though his story and life were really sad since he had no control when these things happened, and his wife was finally fed up and left him. Our medications at that time were primitive at best, although I'm not sure when lithium became available.

We were encouraged to mix with the patients to see how they interacted, and one evening when I had night duty, I decided to go into the day room and see what was happening. Most of the patients were there watching television and were very quiet, but things got really weird when an ad came on and no one moved. I began to realize that between their medications and their illnesses, there was practically no normal human interaction. After that I stayed in the locked nurse's station where the residents and nurses stayed most of the time.

One sad story involved a mild-mannered schizophrenic. This man was in his mid-forties and still lived with his parents. He had worked for the postal service for a number of years and would go home at the end of the day and have dinner and watch comedies on TV until bed time. One night his parents came into the room where he was watching TV as usual and laughing, but he'd forgotten to turn the TV on. He told us he'd watched his hallucinations for years until his parents found out and sent him to the VA. He lost his job and now just sat around all day with a disease for which we really had no cure and very poor treatment.

Psych specialists seem to lose many of their medical skills just from nonuse and maybe from noninterest. One day we got a page to the locked unit stat (an abbreviation of *status,* meaning, “right now”), which was very unusual on psych. The resident and I ran up to the ward and got the door open expecting some patient out of control and dangerous. When we got there, we found one of the patients had had a nose bleed and the nurse panicked, but the bleed had been controlled by another patient who was an orthopedic surgeon. This man had just gotten out of residency and gone into practice when World War 2 broke out and he was drafted. He told me he suddenly found himself making less than his insurance fees and with a huge debt for equipment leases and for the expenses of running an office. Apparently he lost control and became violent in basic training and went directly from there to the VA psych ward where he had stayed ever since. That at least is the story he told, but since he wasn’t my patient, I didn’t know the parts he wasn’t telling.

I also drew the VA for my surgery rotation, which I viewed as fortunate because in those days I was a pipe smoker and could buy tobacco cheap at the canteen in the VA as long as I was assigned there. The story about the chief of surgery was that he was an excellent surgeon but had to work at the VA because he threw such tantrums in the OR that nobody in private practice would refer to him because they didn’t want to assist him. One of the junior residents had a scar on his forehead that he swore was from a thrown retractor the chief hit him with when he was a student. The nursing staff kept a backup scrub nurse (the nurse who hands instruments to the surgeon) ready whenever the chief operated because the nurse who started the procedure would frequently leave crying about halfway through the case, and the backup would have to take over and finish up.

There were four students assigned to the ward at a time, and our group worked well together except one guy. When we were assigned to go around and change post op dressings, he was never to be found. It was so consistent we began to refer to him as the Gray Ghost. He would turn up whenever one of the attendings showed up to talk about a case, however, and we could never figure out how he knew and where he hid. He did exactly the same thing at graduation, appearing out of nowhere as we were already marching in.

We had one corpsman as a patient who had been in Vietnam and had been with the marines in the Mekong Delta in the swamps. He had a nasty wound from a bungee stick, a piece of bamboo stuck in the ground with a sharpened point sticking up. The point was frequently smeared with human feces. He had developed an abscess, but he told me it hadn't been a problem until he got sent home because the leaches in the swamp had kept it drained until he came home when the abscess began to grow.

One Friday, we had a SAW (Spanish American War veteran) brought in from the old soldier's home because he'd taken a fall and cut his head. The resident thought this was a great case for a student since the face of a man nearly a hundred years old probably wasn't a great concern if it got a scar, so he put me in a procedure room and told me to sew it up. I knew next to nothing about sewing but set up with sterile drapes and got out the necessary instruments when the man started moving all over the table. I shouted at him to please lie still, thinking he was confused, but when he didn't stop I took the drapes off and found he was convulsing. After convulsions there is a period known as post ictal when the patient is somnolent, so when that happened I finished sewing up his cut and put a dressing on it. I then told the resident what had happened, and it was apparent he would have to be admitted for observation for intracranial bleeding, but it was five on Friday so we took the gurney down to the neurosurgery floor. We left it in front of the nursing desk and went back to our own floor where the resident called the neurosurgery resident and told him there was a SAW on his ward that had a seizure post fall and needed to be admitted for observation. In medicine that is known as a dump and happens fairly frequently.

The chief surgery resident was doing the last year of his residency for the second time, and I hope he wasn't ever allowed to practice surgery because he lacked the confidence to ever do surgery on his own. As chief resident, he was supposed to do his own surgeries, but I remember being a second assistant behind a junior resident when the chief resident was supposed to do a vagotomy. This procedure was to cut the vagus nerve above where it entered the stomach to cause the pylorus (out flow tract of the stomach) to relax and to decrease the acid production. The nerve comes down along the esophagus, and because the esophagus is stretchy and the nerve not so much, it's fairly easy to identify by stretching the esophagus and seeing what fibers bow-string. He couldn't seem to understand how to recognize what was what, and even though the junior resident and I told him where it was, he finally ended up crying, and the attending had to come in and show him where it was.

This level of surgery taking as long as four to five hours to remove a gallbladder put me off on becoming a surgeon, something I regretted later in life. In private practice a good surgeon could usually do a gallbladder in an hour or less (before scopes). The student stood in one place for the entire time, usually holding a retractor and being bored. One of my friends, after working all night, fell asleep on the end of a retractor and fell backward lacerating the liver with his instrument and severely irritating the surgeon.

Since there were no outpatient surgery clinics at the VA, we were posted to the county ER in the evenings some of the time. When you're a student in the ER, the resident tries to give you the easy cases. I remember one of my first cases in the county ER was an old Chinese patient who had come in complaining of a sore toe. I guess the resident figured even a student couldn't screw up a sore toe too badly. The gentleman spoke no English, but when I went in to the exam room, he pointed to the offending toe. When we got the sheets off, it proved to be a great toe, which was absolutely black and becoming gangrenous. On further exam, he proved to have a large pulsating mass in his abdomen. So my first ER case was an abdominal aortic aneurysm with a loss of blood supply to the legs and developing gangrene, hardly the easy case the resident thought but very satisfying to me to be able to make the diagnosis and get the vascular team on the case.

I also learned very early on that the ER is potentially a very dangerous place. I've seen statistics that show that the average in the US is one violent incident per ER per day. I was sitting in the ready room with the other student and a couple of house staff when the admitting clerk asked a man his name to get started filling out his chart. He screamed, "Why do you want to know that?" and knocked her cold. Of course all the house staff and students immediately surrounded the man, and the psych resident finally talked him down. We learned later the family had brought him in because he was a paranoid schizophrenic who had stopped taking his medications.

The students and residents at the county had developed a system of points (called gomer points) to indicate how bad an admission was. You got five points if the admitting orders started with "bath stat" and another five points if the orders ended with "sorry.". If the attending surgeon refused to operate, it was worth five points, ten points if the surgical resident refused, and fifteen points if the surgical intern refused. It was worth five points if the patient was found in bed with another patient, ten points if the other patient was of the same sex. Each year the list got longer as students and house staff worked on it.

The bath stat order was not really a joke. We used it frequently with some of the street people. We had a special team consisting of an orderly and a nurse's aide who would take the patient to a special room that had a tub on a pedestal called the bird bath. They would glove up and take the patient's clothes and throw them in the incinerator. They would put the patient into the tub and use a pressure hose and scrub brushes until he was clean. When the patients left the hospital, they would be given clean clothes provided by one of the charities.

The other high point of the surgery rotation was getting free lunches while meeting with the dietician. The lunches were therapeutic lunches composed of diets, such as low sodium or low fat, we would order for the patients. These proved to be so unpalatable most of us started to bring our lunches and ate them after the dietician left.

The other main rotation in the third year was pediatrics. This rotation was always dreaded because you usually spent the whole rotation sick with the various viruses the kids gave you in the clinic. Peds can be fun because the kids are cute, but it can also be the saddest rotation because they are kids and kids aren't supposed to die.

Soon after I started peds, a little girl was admitted with leukemia, which in those days was almost universally fatal. It turned out I earlier had met her father who was a local drug company representative. Shortly after being admitted, she went into leukemic crisis, which is usually the terminal event, and the only way we had to fight it was high dose steroids, which sometimes worked. I sat up all night with that girl, and fortunately her crisis broke with the steroids, but I heard later she died after a few weeks.

One of the other students had a nearly career-ending episode while on pediatrics. He'd seen a six-month old baby brought to the clinic with a high fever and stiff neck. Because this appeared clinically to be meningitis, the student was assigned to do a lumbar puncture to obtain fluid for culture, so we'd know what antibiotic would work best. This is a dangerous procedure in the face of serious infection because the pressure in the brain may be up, and when you remove fluid from the spinal cord, the fluid from the brain can't migrate down fast enough, and the pressure can push the brain into the spinal canal, killing the patient. The student was aware of this and therefore used the smallest spinal needle they had, but in spite of his precautions, the fluid spurted out the top of the manometer (device for measuring intra spinal pressure) before he could pull the needle out and the infant immediately died. All of us on peds were required to go to the autopsy of this baby, including the student who had done the LP. We didn't see him again for three days, and he told me later he almost dropped out of medical school over the incident even though the attendings said he'd done everything right and had just been unlucky.

One night I was in the peds ER when a three-week-old baby was brought in by some newly adoptive parents. The infant was coughing and having trouble breathing. The exam was compatible with pneumonia, but in addition, this infant had a strange appearance and the resident thought he knew what was going on. We took the child to a dark room where the resident put a bright flashlight to the baby's head, and we could see half the head lighted. There was no brain in half the cranium. The adoptive parents had been told the baby was healthy, so the resident decided to tell them only that the child had a severe pneumonia through no fault of theirs and needed to be admitted. The baby was admitted, but no antibiotics were prescribed, and the infant died in a couple days. In those days doctors made decisions like that, but not today. I was just glad it wasn't my decision to make.

Guatemala

When the summer of 1967 came, I finally reaped the rewards of my past two summers working in the Preventive Medicine Department. I got a grant to go to Guatemala with INCAP (the Institute of Nutrition of Central America and Panama), an organization sponsored by the World Health Organization. Sue and I were thrilled, although we were a little worried how we'd live on the $300 a month stipend. Nevertheless, we arranged our airline tickets and got packed and off we went. When we arrived in Guatemala, we were met by a representative of the agency and were whisked through customs with a barely cursory inspection of our luggage.

The agency had arranged an apartment for us, and the next day I went to see the institute and meet my boss for the summer. When we entered the building, I noticed they were sweeping up glass around the front windows and asked my guide what had happened. I was told a Guatemalan senator had lived across the street but had been assassinated the day before with a car bomb. Across the street meant across a wide six-lane boulevard. Nobody but me seemed particularly worried about this. I was given a card with my picture on it, identifying me as working for WHO, which gave me diplomatic immunity. I learned later these were only useful if you could find a policeman who could read.

My boss in the Microbiology Department turned out to be a fairly young Costa Rican with a DSc from Harvard. The department secretary was a multilingual Guatemalan young woman whose father was the regional representative of Oneida Silver. The man I was to work most closely with was a Guatemalan doctor who had done a pediatrics residency in England and had taught pediatrics at a medical school in the US for several years. I was going with him and a team of lab techs and a nutritionist to a field station in the mountains outside Guatemala City. This station had been used in studies by INCAP for years and had a pretty good relationship with the people of the village. I was warned this relationship must be maintained to protect all the work that had been done there in the past.

Living in a foreign country for the first time was an adventure. My wife heard of a supermarket in Guatemala City and she went there to shop. When I came home that night, she was crying because prices were so high she was sure we were going to starve. She went into the kitchen and started dinner when I heard her scream. I rushed to the kitchen to see what had gone wrong and discovered when she had opened the plastic-wrapped chicken she'd bought, she found the chicken's claws and head neatly tucked into the body cavity.

We soon learned that there was a grocery store in the basement of the American Embassy, and since I worked for an international health organization, we were eligible to use it. We also discovered that most of what you needed could be obtained in the Central Market and quite cheaply too. Also in the embassy there was a bulletin board with listings of houses for rent, and we found a very nice two-bedroom house owned by a German woman who worked for the German Trade Association. She was going back to Germany for a sabbatical and needed someone to look after her house and maid. The total price was $130 per month, including the live-in maid and a gardener three days a week. We were also told we could use her car, but looking at the traffic, we were a little afraid to consider that. We rented the house and settled in.

Each day I took the city bus to the institute, and each day about halfway there, the driver would stop in the middle of traffic and grab a bucket from under his seat and run to a fountain and get a bucket of water, which he would pour in the radiator so he could complete his route. Getting to the research station involved loading a van with supplies, three lab techs, the nutritionist, the pediatrician, and me. I was the only non-Guatemalan in the group. Only the pediatrician and the nutritionist spoke any English and I spoke virtually no Spanish.

The institute did have Spanish classes in the late afternoon for those of us who needed them.

There was only one male lab tech and he would always drive. We would stop at a small market on the way where a butcher shop nearly always had a red flag out, meaning they had slaughtered an animal that day and had fresh meat. The butcher would simply wave his hand at what appeared to be a black carcass, and when the black flew away, he would cut off however much you had ordered. There didn't seem to be specific cuts. He'd wrap it in paper and that was our lunch. No one but me seemed to be bothered by the flies.

The trip to the village was always an experience since the Guatemalan lab tech was driving. The route was up a curvy mountain road, which was somewhat narrow, and Guatemalans seemed to never have heard about not passing on curves. We would frequently have to pass three across because either we or someone coming the other way would be passing when we rounded the curve. I was always very relieved when we finally arrived at the village.

The research station was situated next to the central square in the village and had a laboratory, lunch room, and a kitchen where a couple of the village women would cook our lunch. My work station was on a Dutch door because I was examining fresh stool samples on the children, and we didn't have a hood to evacuate the smells. The square next door had a statue and two outhouses. These had all been supplied by the central government and were basically ignored by the Indians. They saw no reason for throwing good night-soil fertilizer into a hole in the ground. The Indians were generally logical if you understood their point of view.

One great example of that came from the village next to ours where a Peace Corps volunteer was teaching school. He came visiting just to speak English awhile and told us a problem he had with a free lunch program. USAID had begun supplying his school with free lunches, which were basically made of US surplus food. They contained a cheese sandwich among other things, and the Peace Corpsman noted the children would open the sandwich and take out the cheese and throw it away and eat the bread. Since much of the reason for the lunches was to increase the protein intake of the kids, he was concerned. When asked why they did this, the children told him there was spoiled cheese in the sandwich because it was yellow. The Indians had never seen yellow cheese, only white, and they feared the yellow would make them sick.

Our mandate was to try to see where the health departments of Central America could get the most for their very limited resources, so INCAP was studying the effects of poor nutrition, frequent infections in the children, and cultural taboos. One thing I noticed was that all the kids were anemic, and our village was at too high an altitude for hookworm, which was abundant on the coast and commonly caused anemia there. The assumption was that these kids were anemic because of their poor diet, which consisted almost entirely of black beans and tortillas. I asked why not test to see if they were losing blood in their stools since I had fresh stools brought in by the mothers each day. My boss agreed, and I began testing each sample for occult (too small an amount to see) blood. We were totally surprised to discover that 95 percent of the stools had blood in them. Since we knew that the average kid got only nine grams of meat on average daily, therefore diet was not contributing to the blood and it had to be coming from the kids. I assumed that it was due to the large parasite loads they were carrying, causing inflammation of the gut.

One of my duties was to go around the village with the pediatrician and get blood samples, from the kids, which we would use to do antibody studies back at the main laboratory. This was not easy because the Indians were terrified of blood so a plan had been devised to take a 250 ml bottle of IV sugar water with us. The Indians had noted that when you got really sick, you would be put in the hospital in Guatemala City and you always got an IV. They had concluded this was very strong medicine. We would get them to agree to allow us to stick the child's finger in return for the bottle of IV fluid, which they would then spoon-feed to the child. It turned out there were IV parlors in the city where they could go and get a liter of fluid IV to make them strong. I have no idea how sterile these were.

Once we got the parents' permission, I would squat down in the dirt floor of the hut to get below the worst of the smoke, stick a screaming three-year-old's finger, and collect the blood with a large capillary tube. If I didn't get good bleeding the first time, there really was no second chance as the parents would have panicked by then.

As we went around the village, I noticed a part of the population was missing and asked the pediatrician where the girls between the ages of about ten and sixteen were. He told me they were hiding because I wasn't from the village, and they couldn't be seen by a male not from their village. Indeed, they couldn't talk with a male even from their village without a chaperone. He told me of a girl who had been caught talking to a man without a chaperone. She had been kicked out of the village as being a prostitute. Of course since she had no way to make a living this became a self-fulfilling prophecy when she was forced to go to the city. Most of the girls were married by sixteen and therefore could deal with non-village males.

One day as we were making our rounds of the village, an elderly lady stopped us, and the pediatrician told me it was her birthday and she wanted us to share a birthday tortilla with her. We entered her hut and squatted down while she gave each of us a rolled tortilla hot off the rock by her fire. When I bit into it, trying to ignore the fact it had been made by a lady who probably had never used hand soap, I bit down on something that I thought had broken my tooth. I tried to keep smiling and asked the pediatrician what was in the tortillas. He said she'd put rock salt in to flavor them because she was too poor to have anything else. While we carefully ate our tortillas, she dug into a chest and brought out her prized possessions, which were black-and-white photos of her family. There were photographers who went to festivals and took pictures for fifty cents with a big old camera with a billow on the front, which he would shoot by taking the lens cap off and counting to ten. This gave me an idea. We brought two cameras with us, one of which was a Polaroid and I used the Polaroid color picture to barter with the Indians so I could take almost any 35 mm picture I wanted. Both of us would end up happy with the trade.

I had to go back to the city earlier than the ,others for my Spanish lessons, so I would walk up to the highway and flag down one of the country buses, most of which were old US school buses. The Guatemalans filled these to the gills and carried passengers' bags and other effects on the roof. There were two men with the bus, a driver, and a conductor who would store things on the roof. Sometimes there were animals such as chickens, which couldn't go on the roof, so they rode with the passengers. The bus had seats that nearly met in the middle, and I soon learned that when the regular seats were full, you were expected to sit in the aisle with one cheek on each side. One of the lady lab techs would drive me from the village to the highway bus stop, but one day we arrived just as the bus left. She was not bothered by this but simply got out of the car and flagged down the next car on the highway going my way and explained to the driver where I needed to go, and he agreed to take me. I rode into the city with him, although he spoke no English and I spoke almost no Spanish, so we just sat silently.

There was a constant security problem because of some Castro guerillas in the hills who would come into the city and shoot up police stations. At night we were told if we had to drive anywhere, we should turn our dome lights on so we could be seen and we wouldn't be shot at. The police were always heavily armed and looked more like marines going into combat than police. They wore helmets and flak jackets and were armed with both pistols and submachine guns. They usually traveled with four officers in a car and two cars, one behind the other, so they could cover the lead car in an ambush. They were fairly free with the use of the weapons as well. One day one of the other Americans at the institute was walking down the street when he heard gunfire nearby. Naturally he and everybody around him dived for cover, but when he looked out, all that had happened was a motorcyclist had started down the wrong way on a one-way street and a cop on the corner had fired his weapon into the air to attract his attention. The motorcyclist simply turned and rode off and the cop put his gun away.

The guerillas would park a car across from a police station and then bring a second car down the street and throw a grenade in the front door of the station; when the police came running out, the men in the parked car would machine gun them. As a consequence, there were always two policemen sitting on the front porch of the station with submachine guns. Our Guatemalan friends told us to always cross the street rather than walk in front of the police station because you could get caught in a cross fire. We also noticed the same was true of policemen just walking around town, and even in crowds at the zoo there was a bubble of empty space around the officers because nobody wanted to stand too near.

Castro tried to get the Indians on his side, and one technique he tried was to drop crystal radios from planes, which could only receive Radio Havana. We were told this had happened just before we got there, but there were no radios anywhere because the American tourists had bought them all up as curiosities. Apparently we weren't the only ones who didn't understand.

The laws of Guatemala were based on the French system where you are guilty until you prove your innocence. There was a bulletin board in the US Embassy, in an area where only Americans could go, which had the official recommendation that if you were in an accident, you should run. There was an American pathologist working at Guatemala General Hospital who disappeared one day and nobody could find him. His brother worked in our institute and decided his brother must have been picked up by the police, so he went to the central jail and he never came back. The families hired a Guatemalan lawyer and he got them both out. All that had happened was the pathologist saw his car get hit in the hospital's parking lot. He'd called the police and went out to confront the motor scooter driver who had hit him. However, the police were there first, and when he got there, the motor scooter was driving off and the police arrested him instead. He ended up in a tank with murderers, thieves, and everybody else until he was rescued.

I was nearly arrested because my wife had her birthday while we were there, and her parents sent her some money in the mail. When the mail got to us there, was one dollar and the birthday card in the envelope. We were surprised there was any money left but didn't think much about it. A couple days later, I got a note that we had a package waiting at the central post office, which we assumed was another birthday present. Since I was in the field all day, I gave the note to the institute's messenger and asked him to pick up the package. When I got back that evening, he met me and told me the room where the package was supposed to be was in fact the office of the postal police. It seems that not only is it illegal to send money in the mail, but the person to whom it is addressed can be arrested for it. They were waiting for me to come in, so they could arrest me. The institute had convinced them I had diplomatic immunity, and it was all cleared up by the time I got back to town.

One of the highlights of our trip was a flight to the Mayan ruins at Tikal. This ancient Mayan site is in the jungle of the lowlands of Guatemala and could only be reached by air or by a three-day donkey trip through the jungle. The plane that was to take us there was a vintage DC3 and I had to question its upkeep. When we were to get aboard, I saw rubber hanging from the tire. I could also see the pilot doing his preflight, which seemed to consist of crossing himself. We managed to get to Tikal without incident and landed on a jungle airstrip, which was a place where the larger trees had been knocked down by a bulldozer. Our guide was from Belize and spoke fluent English and French as well as Spanish. He'd worked for years assisting the archeologists from the University of Pennsylvania who were mainly responsible for the excavations. He told us we were lucky to get such a cool day (only about 100° F and 90 percent humidity).

After a full day of climbing around the ruins and using up untold rolls of film, we were again assembled at the runway to await our plane. The plane had taken the seats out and gone for a load of supplies for the archeologists. When they landed, they skidded across the runway nearly clipping a tree with a wing and slid to a stop in front of us. After unloading the supplies and reinstalling the seats, they expected us to get on for the trip back to Guatemala City. I didn't care too much for the plane, but I loved the ancient Mayan history and have followed that interest since.

A few days after a trip to the West Coast, I broke into a high fever. My wife called my boss at the institute, and he recommended a group of three internists, all of whom had done their residencies at Mass General. When one of them saw me, he put me into a private hospital. (Guatemala General was notorious for people not dying of what they were admitted for but what they got while there). Because my fever was so high and we had just returned from the coast, they thought I might have caught malaria. The best time to find the malaria organism in the blood is when the fever goes up, so every time my temperature rose, several lab techs would come rushing in to draw blood and make smears. It soon became apparent I had hepatitis A. The only prevention for this at that time was a shot of gamma globulin, and the institute hadn't recommended it with our other immunizations because they were mostly Central Americans. Hepatitis A was considered a childhood illness there because it was so prevalent. Children don't get nearly as sick as adults with this disease.

I was kept in the hospital for several days. Fortunately, our German landlady was bilingual, and my wife found a complete collection of Ian Fleming's James Bond books, which were the only English books around. I was quite nauseated but they wanted me to eat, so when they brought a menu around I sort of picked things at random. I knew which were meats, vegetables, and drinks, but didn't really care what they were until one day they brought dinner, and I took the metal cover off the plate and found myself looking at a large beef tongue. That didn't help the nausea one bit. I did find I could eat the ice cream even though it had ice crystals in it. It turned out that a private room in this private hospital was $15 a day and even my student insurance paid $25.

After I got out of the hospital, I rested at the rented house for a few days. When the doctor thought I was up to traveling, we had to decide what to do. I really wasn't up to working, but the institute said I could work in the library. Sue had to go back to the United States because she had a teaching job, which started soon, so we decided I might as well go back too. We had bought a number of souvenirs and realized we were going to be overweight with our luggage, so we changed our tickets from TWA to the Guatemalan Airline, Aveoteca. TWA allowed twenty-two pounds per person in luggage and Aveoteca allowed twenty-two kilograms. This meant we were only a few pounds overweight. We had bought a handmade chest, and it had come with a crate built to fit. We put all our purchases in the chest and locked it up thinking it would make things easier in customs if they were all together.

When we arrived for our flight, the agent didn't want to take the chest, telling me it wasn't luggage, but after some wrangling by our institute representative, we convinced him it was our luggage and we saw it go into the cargo hold before boarding. We flew across the gulf to New

Orleans in a DC6, which bounced all across the sky. In the back of the plane there was a man with a parrot on his shoulder. They served dinner, which consisted of some sort of greasy rice and meat dish in a cardboard box with grease soaked through. Since I was still not totally well, I skipped the experience.

When we arrived in New Orleans, it was about midnight and we couldn't believe how hot it was. The approach had been beautiful because of the shrimp boats with bright lights over their nets to attract the shrimp. When we went to collect our luggage, the chest wasn't there; it apparently had been removed after we got on the plane. There was a long holdup while the customs agent screamed at the man with the parrot. Parrots and similar birds can carry parrot fever (psittacosis), which can be life threatening, and parrots are subject to prolonged quarantine to keep it out of the country. After clearing customs we went to the Aveoteca counter and the agent there found our chest still in Guatemala and agreed to get it to the States and walk it through customs for us. I gave him the key to the chest. That was the last time I saw that key.

When we got back home, we had $10 between the two of us to live the rest of the month, but we survived. I arranged with the medical school to do a preceptorship with a GP near our home since part of the time we were to be in Guatemala was to have been my senior elective time, and I had to get a grade to graduate. A couple weeks after we got back, we got a call from US customs in Seattle that our chest had arrived in bond, and we needed to come down and take it through customs. Aveoteca again failed to keep their promise but at least they'd sent our stuff back. I explained to the customs agent what had happened and he was very sympathetic. I had a list of everything in the chest, and he looked it over and said we were over our limits, and since the chest was considered furniture, which had the lowest tariff, he charged me $2 and let it go. That, of course, was before drugs were such a problem. I had to pick the lock when we got home, but everything was there.

I learned that I liked tropical medicine and loved working with the people but felt a lifetime of working with the governments of these countries would eventually drive me crazy. I decided to look at another specialty.

My rotation in the GP's office was ideal because he didn't care if I had to go home and rest part of the time. The office was a typical suburban office, and the patients were very nice as a whole. One elderly lady came in for follow-up on her blood pressure and the physician wasn't watching the manometer as he pumped it up. These devices used mercury for the measurement, and when I looked at the device mercury was coming out the top. The physician was still listening for the pulse to stop and hadn't realized the pressure was above 300 mm Hg, which was as high as the device went. This is called "lead pipe syndrome" and occurs when the arteries have lost so much elasticity that the pressure, when the heart contracts, shoots up much higher than it would when the arteries are springy.

We had one incident where a sixteen-year-old female needed a pelvic exam for some reason. Because she was very anxious, the physician asked his assistant and me to wait outside the room while he did the exam (I felt leaving his female assistant outside was a mistake and I still do). After a couple of minutes we heard him yelling for help, and when we entered the room found the young lady had panicked and had her legs wrapped around his head in a death grip. Trying to keep straight faces, the assistant and I unwrapped her legs and got her to settle down. I never did decide whether the red face on the physician was due to strangulation or embarrassment.

This experience in primary care confirmed my interest in exploring general practice further. In spite of the university's prejudice, I felt I would keep an open mind toward general practice.

The Final Year

Our Ob-Gyn training started the fourth year and was split between the University Hospital and the County Hospital with a switch in the middle since they had entirely different populations. My group started at the university for our first four weeks and had very little in the way of lectures before going right on the ward. I arrived on the ward early in the morning and found no one at the nurses' station. I could hear activity down the hall, so I decided just to wait until someone could tell me my duties. In those days women were prepped with a pubic shave and enema when they came in in labor. Someone had the idea that these procedures would decrease the incidence of neonatal infection. As I was sitting there, the door to a prep room across the hall opened, and a nurse stuck her head out and shouted "Doctor, I need you in here right now." I looked around, but there was no one else in the area, and she shouted "you" and pointed at me. I went into the prep room to find a lady lying on the prep table with the perineum covered with shaving cream and a tiny head appearing at the vagina. As I got to the bottom of the table, she gave a huge push and the infant came squirting out. Newborns are always slippery since they're wet, but when you add shaving cream and panic they're really hard to hang on to. I managed to corral the little squirt and get him wrapped in a blanket. I had no idea what to do with the afterbirth, but the resident showed up about that time and took over. I had done my first delivery about ten minutes after reporting for duty!

Because of the nature of OB, we were expected to sleep in the hospital every other night and be available for routine deliveries. This soon resulted in a lot of sleep deprivation to the point that one morning we were making rounds on the previous night's deliveries when the resident asked one of the students how a particular delivery had gone, and the student had no recall of having done a delivery. He had apparently done the whole thing while asleep.

Most deliveries at that time were done with an episiotomy, which is a cut in the posterior vagina either in the midline or off to one side. The conventional wisdom was that this prevented excessive stretching, which would result in the bladder falling into the vagina later in life.

Obviously, if you made such a cut, it would have to be repaired after the delivery.

We were warned to keep our needle parallel with the floor of the vagina to avoid getting into the rectum. We were required to do a rectal exam after completing a repair to be sure we hadn't gotten into the rectum. My first repair was about two in the morning, and after finishing, I dutifully checked and found suture bowstringing across the inside of the rectum with every stitch. I had to take the entire repair down and start again. I took until 4:00 a.m. to finally get it right. I never did that again.

We had one professor who was apparently considered very handsome and who had a certain number of private patients. When one of his patients came in, he would turn up in the dressing room to put on a scrub suit and then spent considerable time in front of a mirror adjusting his cap until it had just the right jaunty level. He never gowned but simply stood at the head of the table and talked with the patient while the resident and med student did the actual delivery. The women were so mesmerized by him they had no idea who delivered their babies. This same attending had the same ability in clinic where two or three medical students would practice pelvic exams on one woman while he talked to them.

There was one story that went around the floor, which I suspect was an urban legend, about an elderly attending physician who insisted on doing his own deliveries and who dropped one baby into the kick bucket at the end of the table when it slipped through his fingers. When he went to pick it up, it slipped again and again landed in the bucket. When he picked it up again and got good control, he commented to the mother, "Sometimes I have to drop them three times to get them breathing."

One day an Asian lady newly arrived was brought in for an initial OB exam. She had had one child previously by C-section, so it was presumed we would repeat it this time. She was obviously scared, and as I did her exam, every time I'd turn to get a different instrument, she'd grab the sheet and curl up into a little ball. I'd have to sort of straighten her out for each step in the exam, so I was fairly certain there was no chance I'd get her to cooperate with the pelvic. So I went out and found our only female resident (today most of the OB residents are female) and asked her to try. She came in and tried to get the young woman to allow her to do the exam but with absolutely no success. The resident said we didn't need to know the pelvis size since it would be a repeat C-section anyway, and the patient never did get a pelvic. Because pregnancy accelerated cervical cancer, we needed a Pap smear, but she was just going to have to take her chances.

IUDs were just coming into vogue, and we were taught to place them in the uterus in clinic. The university was experimenting with one that was made of metal and looked like a group of paper clips strung together into a spring side by side. This was compressed and introduced into the uterus where it would spring open and stick into the uterine walls. This resulted in severe cramping and the patients could rarely tolerate it and it never made it to market.

During the day we had lectures on both OB and Gyn and I suppose helped in surgery but those surgeries were so boring I really can't remember them specifically. Usually the med student got to hold a retractor to hold tissue out of the surgeon's field of view. With the vaginal hysterectomy this meant sort of leaning over the back of the surgeon for hours without even being able to see what he was doing.

After our time at the University Hospital our team moved to the county hospital where OB was an entirely different kettle of fish. Upon arrival the first morning, we were told the resident and intern had been in the delivery rooms for thirty-six hours straight, so the other two medical students were each given a delivery room and went right to work so the house staff could go to sleep. I was assigned to a ward full of high-risk pregnancies. There were several cases of pre-eclampsia and one of hyper emesis gravidarum. Pre-eclampsia and eclampsia are very dangerous disorders, which consist of high blood pressure and eventually convulsions. The mother's reflexes get faster and faster until when you do a reflex the limb keeps bouncing (clonus). At that point convulsions are about to occur. The treatment available was magnesium sulfate by IV until delivery could be accomplished, which definitively treated the condition. The resident told me to just go around the room, and when clonus occurred to push more magnesium sulfate. After I'd started, the nurse objected to a medical student doing this, so I gave her the choice of waking the resident or doing it herself. She decided to let me go ahead. If the point of convulsions was reached, the baby usually died as did half the mothers, so this was not an insignificant threat. By definition once convulsions start, it is no longer pre-eclampsia but has become true eclampsia. In my career, I have seen only two eclamptics and both arrived in the ER convulsing and both babies died as did one mother.

Hyperemesis gravidarum is like morning sickness on steroids. In the past these mothers would die from malnutrition and even today frequently require hospitalization and IV fluids and nutrition. For the one lady I had with hyperemesis management was simply a matter of keeping her IV fluids balanced.

One of the things you learned at the county hospital was to do what you had to, to keep the patient going. Most of the nurses were very helpful and pragmatic, allowing the students to do what was necessary, but we had one old harridan who thought her job was to protect the patients from us. On one occasion a medical student arrived out of breath to get a newborn Ambu (breathing bag) because they had an infant coding in the ER. This silly woman tried to take it from him because it was supposed to remain on the OB unit even though we had no cases that looked like it would be needed in the next few minutes. Since there was no time to argue with her, I simply grabbed the bag and handed it to the med student and told him to run while I stood in front of the nurse. When the resident finally caught up with what had happened, he agreed there was no excuse to let a baby die over a regulation. After that I had no further problems with that nurse.

One of the things we learned while on OB was circumcision. I never liked that procedure as it was practiced at that time. We were told it didn't hurt the baby, but I wondered why they screamed bloody murder when you did it. The procedure was done with no anesthetic of any kind and involved crushing tissue and sticking safety pins through the skin. Whoever thought that was painless was nuts.

We had some excitement during my OB rotation at the county hospital when the queen of the gypsies arrived to be admitted to labor. I have since learned that there are no king and queen of the gypsies, but the gypsies will use this designation sometimes when dealing with non-gypsies. The group set up camp right on the hospital lawn and moved in. The hospital was frantic because there were gypsies wandering all over and things were starting to disappear. The baby was delivered, and the child and mother were discharged as quickly as it was felt safe to do so, much to the relief of the administrators of the hospital.

I learned a lesson in the clinic at the county that stood me in good stead later. We had an elderly lady come in for an annual exam, and she was assigned to me. After the breast exam the nurses set her up for the pelvic, and as I sat on the stool, I noticed she had a butterfly tattooed on each buttock. That's when I first realized that old people hadn't always been old and had life stories you might not imagine. We had another lady who had been a prostitute who had "sweet" tattooed on one breast and "sour" on the other.

One very strange OB case was presented at rounds. This was a young pregnant girl who eventually died because the real problem wasn't recognized until too late. The girl had come to the ER complaining of chest pain and difficulty breathing. The only significant history was that she had suffered a gunshot wound to her high abdomen and chest a couple years earlier. A chest x-ray showed multiple air-fluid levels (level areas of light below dark showing fluid with air above it). She was admitted with a diagnosis of lung abscesses and started on antibiotics but got progressively short of breath and eventually died. At autopsy it turned out the previous bullet had passed through her diaphragm, and when she had surgery for that, a scar had formed in the diaphragm and under the pressure of pregnancy had ruptured, allowing the gut to migrate into her chest. That was what had been seen on x-ray.

OB was generally a very relaxed and fun field because you usually had positive results. However at that time, we expected to have 5 percent stillbirths. Today OB has become very high tech and tends to have many more worries and in my view is much less fun for the practitioner.

One of the rotations of the fourth year was neurology, and we were kept busy with ward work. Many of the patients were not functional mentally and required various tubes and machinery to maintain life. I had the joy of trying to take a history on a woman on a rocking bed. This was the replacement for the old iron lung and did as its name said, rocked the patient from near upright to slightly inverted thereby allowing gravity to assist her diaphragms to breath. The patient could talk in short phrases as she exhaled and still had to pause for two or three breaths between phrases. One could get quite dizzy watching this patient's head swinging through an arc.

One morning I was making rounds on neurology when we found a patient covered with plaster. The ceiling had given away and landed all over the bed and the patient, but the patient was so far gone he never noticed. The county hospital was always in such poor repair that this sort of incident was not unusual.

Neurology was also the rotation where I learned nurses could do things by themselves. The typical university nurse would call the medical student for various procedures, but one night I had just gotten to bed at about 3:00 a.m. when the nurse called to tell me one of the neurology patients had pulled out his nasogastric tube. I guess I groaned because she asked if I would like her to put it back down. I asked if she could and she just laughed. It seemed she had just started at the county coming from a private hospital, and there they did all that sort of thing. Going back to sleep was just wonderful.

Neurology had another unit in a second part of town where their chronic patients stayed. The resident gave us a sweet old lady to work up, and we took a history from her. She said she'd only been there a couple of days and needed to go home to feed her cats. We were unable to elicit a complaint from her, and she seemed to function pretty well. When we went back to the resident to explain we couldn't figure out why she'd been admitted, he went back with us and started asking the standard mental function questions. We learned it was 1918 and Teddy Roosevelt was president. She was one of the best confabulators I ever saw and was kept on the chronic ward and given to each set of students as they came through. (A confabulator is a person who makes up stories about what is going on because they are confused.)

One of our rotations was outpatient psychiatry. Each student was assigned a couple of patients to try to deal with. I had one lady who came in repeatedly saying her life was so bad she was going to jump. After a couple of sessions I asked if she had ever tried to jump, and she said she had gotten on an overpass railing but got so scared she froze and the fire department had to lift her down. Having heard that, I decided we might get a little farther in her therapy if we got the jumping out of the way, so one day when she said she wanted to jump, I suggested she go ahead. She got up, went into the waiting room, climbed up on a chair and jumped off. She then came back to the room and said she felt much better. This became a ritual we went through at the start of each session thereafter.

My other patient was a young African-American from the ghetto who was always so agitated that he talked a mile a minute and used primarily ghetto terms so that I figured I understood about 20-30 percent of what he said. It was a revelation that this young man had grown up in this country, but his speech was such that I couldn't understand him. We discussed this and he continued to be agitated but was able to use words I understood if he concentrated.

One day one of the psychiatric attendings took us to the psych ward at the county hospital. All the patients there were untreated. They were brought in by families or police for evaluation and placement. After evaluation they would be parceled out to the state hospital or the VA or other facilities. The psychiatrist we were with was a small woman. There were two women and two men in the student group. We were taken to an interview room on the psych ward (which was of course locked), and one of the attendants brought in the patient to be interviewed. This proved to be a heavily muscled, largish man who allegedly had been brought in by the police when they picked him up with a Luger on his way to kill his mother because she said something on the phone that angered him. As the interview progressed, it turned out he had been a marine and had three tours in Vietnam when he was sent back during his third tour because he had become "kill crazy," which apparently meant he'd quit differentiating between friend and foe. After he came back and was given a dishonorable discharge, he was involved in a major car accident and sustained severe injury to the frontal lobe of his brain. What this meant basically was whatever control he had of himself was gone. As the story progressed, the psychiatrist became increasingly pale and the other male student and I exchanged glances thinking we couldn't handle him if he suddenly went off. The patient told us he wanted to go back to Vietnam because he loved shooting those little animals (Vietnamese). When he was put back into his locked cell, the psychiatrist said she was going to recommend that he be locked up at the state psychiatric facility for the criminally insane. The problem, as she explained it to us, was that he could only be held for ninety days and then had to be released, even though we all knew it was only a matter of time until he killed someone. The law had been pushed through by well-intentioned people who had absolutely no understanding.

One of the high points of the senior year was the matching program. This was how one got an internship (today called a first year residency). Basically, we were given a list of hospitals looking for house staff and we picked our top choices. Naturally we wanted to see the facilities so most of us spent Christmas break visiting hospitals. I had found a couple interesting openings in California and visited one in Sacramento, which was so bad the ambulances were leaving the ER with their lights and sirens on. I distinctly remember an intern in the hallway with a drunk from a car accident trying to put a chest tube into the man and the man cheering him on yelling, "Push harder, Doc, push harder."

I had also thought about changing the scenery entirely and seeing if medicine was practiced differently in other parts of the country, so I arranged to see several internships in the Midwest and the East. Since my wife's parents lived in the Midwest, this worked out well. She could stay with them and we could have Christmas at their place. I traveled to a number of hospitals but wasn't really wild about any of them. After Christmas, I decided to see if I could interview at a hospital nearby, which was one of the local university's facilities. That turned out to be the best place I'd seen the whole trip. We went back to home, and I set up my list with one of the Sacramento hospitals first and the Midwest hospital second.

Another fourth year rotation was in urology, and I was again posted at the VA. This had good and bad aspects. We had lots of material from the older vets but very little female pathology. Far and away the most common procedure was the TURP, which stands for transurethral resection of the prostate. I learned early on that this wasn't the simple procedure it was sometimes cracked up to be. One afternoon I was observing a procedure, which was usually a boring job since we didn't have television monitors in those days, and I couldn't see what the resident was doing, when the patient started convulsing.

The anesthesiologist had no idea what was going on, but when we removed the drapes, the patient's abdomen was massively distended. Apparently the resident had perforated the thin part of the urethra known as the membranous urethra and the irrigation fluid, which is used to wash out the "chips" of prostrate, was able to get into the abdominal cavity and was absorbed. The result was that the patient's sodium was down to 115 (normal 140), and he died.

One day we were making the rounds and found one of the post-op patients had not been keeping his catheter clean and the nurse gave him an ultimatum that either he must wash it or she would. She left him a basin of soapy water and a wash cloth and we continued rounds. We finished rounds and were sitting at the nurse's desk writing orders for the day when that patient came out of the room and started down the hall holding his catheter out in front of him pulling his anatomy straight out in extreme pain. He had thought the nurse meant to wash the whole catheter and had tried to pull it out. These are held in by a balloon on the end, which needs to be deflated to remove them, but he knew nothing of this, so he had gotten the balloon about halfway down his penis where it stuck, causing him a lot of pain. To complicate matters a candy striper was delivering a chart, and she met him in the middle of the hall. They did a little dance back and forth to get by each other with the girl looking at the ceiling the whole time trying not to look at his catheter and attached appendage. She finally got past him and ran down the hall, and we never saw her again. When we stopped laughing, we changed the man's catheter and he went back to bed.

We had one patient with fascinating stories who was getting a drain in his scrotum. He'd been stationed in the Philippines where he'd contracted elephantiasis. This is a disease caused by a tiny worm, which can be in such massive numbers they block the lymphatic drainage to a limb or organ. In his case they blocked the drainage from his scrotum, which at one point had reached the size of a watermelon. At this point the scrotal contents had simply liquefied and had had to be drained out. He had stories about being a fishing boat captain. Unfortunately, he had started drinking with his customers, and after a while, he was drinking with or without customers. Eventually he said he'd tried to park his fishing boat in downtown and that was the end of the charter business. He told me he'd reached the point of drinking two-fifths of rum daily. He was a big man but that approaches the largest intake I've ever encountered.

One day we got a stat call to the general outpatient clinic. While the VA did not have an ER (now called an ED since it's no longer a room but a department,) it did have two older physicians whose judgment was frequently questionable. When we arrived there, we found a SAW (Spanish American War veteran) sent in by the old soldiers home with florid congestive heart failure. He had foam coming from his mouth and was barely breathing. The urology resident panicked as he couldn't remember what to do, so he put me in charge of starting resuscitation while he contacted the medicine resident. The treatment in those days was rotating tourniquets to trap blood in the extremities and morphine to relax the patient. When the medicine resident got there, we left him to take care of the man. The urology resident asked the doctor in the outpatient clinic why he had called urology, and the indignant answer was that the patient had a catheter therefore it was clearly a urology case, which was as silly as saying he had false teeth so he was clearly a dental case.

We had just gotten in a new drug that was very helpful in congestive heart failure but was only at the county hospital under study protocols and required permission of the chief of medicine to use. This was a very powerful diuretic (causes you to lose fluid) to lower the fluid overload these people had. We tried it on an elderly lady who came in in similar condition to my man at the VA, and it was amazing how quickly she improved. However, when we made rounds the next day and the resident was bragging about how well this drug worked, we asked her how she felt and the response was "What?" It turned out that this drug occasionally attacked the auditory nerves and left the patient deaf. In spite of this danger, it was released and was on the market for several years because of its strongly positive effects. It was eventually replaced by a similar drug called Lasix (furosimide), which is still in widespread use today and does not cause deafness.

Our senior year we also rotated through renal clinic, which included hypertension and fluid balance. This was a big deal because the chief of Medicine and the chief at the County were both renologists. The chief demonstrated his prodigious memory when he called on me to answer a question as to the most likely organism in a urinary infection. He'd asked me a similar question 2 years before during chief's rounds, and then I had to guess between two answers and got it right. This time I also could narrow it to two organisms and guessed again. He looked at me and said, "Andrews, that's twice you've guessed right." He remembered my answer from two years previously, out of all the students in the school.

The fluid balance team consisted of three students and one medicine resident. We had to arrive at the hospital at four each morning in order to have all the testing done and the orders written before the regular medicine types started their rounds. All the fluids the patient passed the day before (urine and gastric juice from a nasogastric tube primarily) were kept under the bed, and we were required to measure the potassium loss from the previous day, so we could replace it. Many of these patients were very difficult because they were in renal failure. In those days we didn't do kidney transplants and there were only a limited number of dialysis machines. We tried to keep patients alive as long as possible in case there was an opening on one of the machines, and the God Committee chose them. The God Committee was supposedly made up of a mixture of clergy, physicians, and ethicists and decided who was worthy enough to get one of the precious slots on a machine. The members were a secret and the criteria they used were not available to the public.

We then stumbled through the day and went to lecture and clinic until 5:00 p.m. when we raced home to get to bed before the next day started. Much of what we did was very discouraging because we only had three or four drugs for high blood pressure and they tended to have very nasty side effects. I distinctly remember one very obese African-American baker who had severe high blood pressure and could only be controlled with a drug called guanethidine. The problem was that when his blood pressure was controlled, it dropped out of sight whenever he stood up, so he was totally non-functional.

We also were exposed to some of the specialties in short bursts. We would go to the dermatology clinic at the end of the day, and they would take us from room to room in the clinic where they had saved some of the most interesting patients from the clinic that day. One day they presented a scroungy-appearing man with a diffuse rash, which was worse in his armpits and groin. He was homeless and had been sleeping under a bridge. As we had crowded into the clinic room, one of the students had sat on a vacant chair because we had been on our feet all day, but he stood up very suddenly when the resident told us the diagnosis was lice. He realized he was sitting on the man's clothes which had been draped on the chair. He didn't pick any up but he itched for a week anyway.

For cardiology I was assigned to a private cardiologist in the downtown area. He was older and had been a charter member of the Board of Cardiology. I followed him when he made rounds in the hospital as well as observing him in his office in one of the big downtown office buildings. He seemed to make most of his living reading ECGs for insurance companies. He also did a number of two-step tests (the predecessor to the treadmill test) in his office. When I was with him, he admitted a patient with new onset atrial fibrillation (irregular heart beat because the rhythm centers in the atria have lost control) but didn't know how to do electrocardioversion and simply pushed quinadine until the patient either converted to normal rhythm or started to vomit (sign of toxicity of the drug). Even in those days he was ten years out of date, and I began to suspect he hadn't learned any new techniques since he got his board certification.

I did get to observe some more modern techniques at University Hospital where they were starting to do cardiac catheterization (placing a hollow tube into the heart through the vessels and injecting x-ray dye while under a fluoroscope). A patient had arrested in the emergency room, and they had managed to resuscitate him and took him to the cath lab to see if there was anything that could be surgically repaired. While on the table his heart slowed radically, and they pushed some adrenaline (epinephrine) and the effects were amazing. The heart sped up and began contracting so hard it looked like a wash rag being rapidly wrung out. Unfortunately the problem turned out to be a massive pulmonary embolus (blood clot to the lung), and even today, such patients can seldom be resuscitated, and he proceeded to die.

The senior year always ended with a program put on by the seniors, which included roasts of some of the more prominent faculty. Much preparation went into this and it was performed *after* grades were out. Our ventriloquist got the chief to sit on his lap like a dummy and proceeded to characterize him. I was surprised he took it so well. We had an orthopedic surgeon from Australia who had a favorite saying "Payne, you haven't had payne until you've had this." Some of the class had taken a picture of a penis with a ninety-degree bend in it and superimposed a fractured chicken bone over it and played a recording of the professor saying, "Payne, you haven't had payne until you've had this."

There was also the annual awards of the golden, silver, and bronze condoms for the three biggest Pr—in the faculty. These seemed coveted by some of the faculty.

The grand finale for the year was to take the second part of the National Boards. These were much feared, but I thought they were easier than the first part. We had one student who really only wanted to be a pediatric psychiatrist and didn't see the reason for taking all these other subjects. He took gynecology three times before they passed him (just barely), and he was called into the dean's office and told they would pass him and allow him to graduate him if he passed the second part of the boards. He had the lowest score in the class, but our school was such that he ended up in the upper third in the country and was allowed to graduate.

Finally, all eighty of us received our diplomas, took our Hippocratic oaths, and were ready to move on to more training in our respective fields.

Internship

In the spring of my senior year I received notice that I had matched at the hospital in the Midwest, so after graduation, we got ready to move. Traditionally, internship starts on July 1 each year, so we had a few weeks to move. A friend of mine was informed the morning of matching that he hadn't matched because after picking his internships, he had gone for a visit and removed all but one from his list. That was the most popular internship on the West Coast. Early the morning of matching he was called into the dean's office where they had a list of internships around the country that hadn't filled, and he and the dean got on the phone. He selected the US Public Health Service Hospital in New Orleans, which was part of the Tulane University system. He and his wife had never lived beyond the West Coast, but they dutifully pulled a U-Haul to New Orleans and arrived just before July 1. After one day, he decided no one could live in that climate and pulled his U-Haul back to home where he was able to find an internship in a private hospital. He was their only native English-speaking intern.

My internship was at a large private hospital, and we were paid $500 a month, so we weren't going to get rich, but our apartment was supplied in an apartment building right next to the hospital. We had access to a lake across the street and were allowed to bring our families to dinner at the hospital on Sunday night where they always had a choice of a full turkey or a ham dinner. They also supplied my "whites" (we wore white pants, shirts, and a short white coat). The whites were washed and starched in the hospital laundry, which meant they came with so much starch you could lean the pants in a corner and they wouldn't fold up. I had to beat them to get my legs into the pant legs.

The hospital itself was fairly old but had a newer wing added. The old section had such things as imported Italian tile, and the two wings were built differently so that some floors had a ramp up and some a ramp down and one floor in the new section didn't connect to the older section at all.

Many of my colleagues were graduates of the University of Michigan, which was located in the relatively small town of Ann Arbor and had excellent training, but because of the smaller population, they had less experience with direct patient care than some of us who trained in urban centers. Because of this, the non-Michigan interns were assigned to the ER rotation first. As an intern, the ER was the best rotation and also the worst rotation. In our hospital the ER rotation was twenty-four hours on and twenty-four hours off. I always found this a difficult schedule to live with since, when you got off work, you wanted to go right to bed, but that meant you would be up for hours before you started your next shift and even more tired after. I usually split the difference and got some sleep when I got home, then staggered around in a stupor and slept before going back to work.

The other rotations were generally thirty-six hours on and twelve hours off. That made things easy because you knew what you were going to do when you were off. When I had interviewed, I had been told we would be on every third day, but that never happened.

In those days we didn't have an ER specialist and most ERs were run by the house staff. Our ER had one intern and nobody else, so the responsibility was great. Many of the attendings would want us to call them about their patients, but much of the time we were just too busy. I do recall one time when I called an attending about his patient who came in with a pelvic infection, which proved to be gonorrhea. I explained I had treated her and her husband and would file the necessary reports with the Health Department. The attending became very upset and told me I had just ruined their marriage. It seems he had known the husband had the disease and had put the wife on an antibiotic (not the recommended one) on some trumped-up diagnosis. I didn't say what I thought of his ethics but told him I had no choice but to do what the law required. Later, when I ran into this attending at the hospital, I asked him what had happened to the couple, and he burst out laughing. It seems the couple had never talked about it because she thought she'd caught it from her boyfriend, and he thought he'd caught it from his girlfriend, and they both preferred to just leave it alone.

During my internship, there was considerable racial strife in this country, and every so often the Black Panthers would show up in our ER with some minor problem. They'd try to intimidate everyone stomping around in their combat boots wearing their black berets. They never wanted to wait their turn to be cared for. Because ERs get to see the great underbelly of society, we had a panic button hidden under the desk, which connected to two police departments since our hospital was on the line between two cities. When the button was pushed, police from one city came straight to the ER entrance, and the ones from the other city came in the front entrance, checked with the hospital operator and then went to the ER by the hospital entrance. So when the button was pushed, police would seem to be coming in every door at once. It was amazing how quiet and polite Black Panthers could get.

Most of the ERs I've worked in kept coffee on for the staff, and we'd willingly share with the police officers who might want some. It was partly a subtle bribe to have them hanging around to keep things quiet. Another ER in the same town I interned in had an officer assigned to sit there just to keep order, and on one occasion he actually used his shotgun in the ER when a group of black militants entered the ER with the intent of shutting all the ERs in town. Reportedly, the first militant to enter the ER had a .45 in his hand, and the officer just fired as he came through the door. When the police found out what was going on, they set traps in the parking lots of the other two hospitals. No one turned up at our hospital, but the other one in town had a group show up, and they were arrested in the parking lot.

There's an old dark joke in medicine that says we get to bury our mistakes. One day I was working in the ER when a man crawled in the door screaming and crying. His complaint was stomach pain. I think his theatrics tainted my judgment, but regardless, I examined him and noticed when he was distracted, his tight abdomen would relax. Because I was uncertain, I asked the senior medicine resident to take a look and he agreed. I now know I shouldn't have told him my suspicions but simply waited on his conclusions. Regardless, we decided to treat him with antacids and sent him home. After shift change, he came back and was admitted for a perforated ulcer. At surgery the anesthesiologist had allowed the blood pressure to drop which caused his kidneys to shut down. The surgical resident decided post op that he needed dialysis and, ignoring the fact he was almost certainly inflamed and forming adhesions, tried to blindly introduce a peritoneal catheter, which perforated several loops of bowel. When taken back to surgery to repair the bowel, the patient died on the table. My original error had set in motion an unbelievable sequence of events, which conspired to kill this patient. I've never forgotten this episode but did learn a number of lessons, which have since stood me in good stead. I learned to try to listen to the patient regardless of how dramatic they are. I also learned not to prejudice my consultant by telling him what I thought before he saw the patient.

Observers are rare in the ER and can be a problem. While I was interning, the administration approved a Swedish high school exchange student, who wanted to go into medicine, to observe for a couple of days. He followed me around and generally was doing fine until a little girl was brought in after being attacked by a dog; she had some terrible wounds on her face. As I was cleaning her wounds and removing dead tissue (debriding), the student said something about needing air and left the trauma room. I saw he was pale and sweating, so I sent my nurse after him, but he'd gone outside and then came back in and proceeded to faint. The nurse was too small to catch him but was able to knock his glasses off his face. He hit face first on the tile floor and broke off his two upper front teeth at the gum line. I had to give him credit when the next day he showed up with two temporaries and stayed for the whole shift.

Another observer incident occurred when I was a resident in the ER. A sheriff's officer brought in a prisoner from the county jail with a pilonidal abscess (an abscess of a cyst that forms over the tail bone and can be quite large). As my nurse and I set up to drain the abscess, I asked the officer to sit in the waiting room. He declined, citing fears the prisoner would run. I told the officer that after what we were going to have to do, this man wasn't running anywhere, but he said he'd been in the worst accidents in the county and wasn't going to have a problem. I proceeded to drain the abscess of about a cup of foul-smelling pus. I heard a noise in the head of the cart and looked up just in time to see the officer's head go below the gurney. When he woke up in the next gurney, we had finished with his prisoner who was still there and going nowhere. I guess car accidents don't generally smell as bad as some pus.

One morning I came on shift to find the intern coming off leaving with his white uniform covered with Betadine and looking like he'd been in a fight. It seems the ambulance had brought in a man who had jumped from a second-story window and was unresponsive. As was protocol, the intern immediately started to place an IV. The man jumped off the cart and pushed the intern into the wall. He then began banging his own head on the tile floor with sufficient force to cause significant damage. Each time the staff tried to stop him, the patient would push them off and return to banging his head. In the process all the IV solutions and supplies on shelves in the room were scattered on the floor so everyone was covered with the solutions. When sufficient force was mustered to control the patient and get him in restraints, it turned out he was a catatonic schizophrenic and thought he was being attacked with the IV needle. He somehow thought he was saving the world by banging his head on the floor. Just one more fun shift in the ER.

One evening we got a call that an ambulance was coming in with a child who had ridden his bike into a barb wire fence and was bleeding profusely. We set up expecting a major arterial wound. The child arrived covered with blood from head to foot, but there was no apparent bleeder. After extensive cleaning we finally found a quarter-inch scalp laceration with a tiny artery squirting away. After a single stitch the "severe bleeding" was controlled and parents and child went home happy.

Ambulance crews have improved in their abilities with training over the years. We got a call one day that an ambulance was en route with a woman in hard labor. A few minutes later a car screeched to a stop in the parking lot, and a man ran in asking where his wife was. It seemed his wife was the woman in the ambulance, and he had beaten them to the hospital. The ambulance came rolling sedately in a few minutes later. They explained they had to stop on the way and deliver the baby. They rolled mother and babe into my exam room, and I checked them both out. Both appeared to be none the worse for the experience except I noticed the baby had a very round head for a newborn; the baby's butt was also very bruised. I cornered the ambulance attendant outside and asked if this was a breech delivery. He didn't know what that was, but when I asked him whether the baby came head first or butt first. He replied, "Butt first, of course." He'd done a breech extraction without even knowing that it was a dangerous presentation.

I had one twelve-year-old brought in moribund. The story was that he'd been having severe diarrhea for several days. The mother told me that the child had always had difficulties with his bowels, and she had used enemas and meds to combat this since infancy. X-rays showed he had large amounts of stool from his splenic flexure (the turn in the colon from the left upper abdomen going down to the rectum) all the way to his rectum. He was having paradoxical diarrhea where the body pushes liquid stool past an obstruction while trying to push the obstruction out. The rectum had a very narrow area visible on x-ray. We had just gotten a multi-twelve lab machine that could do twelve tests at once so I ordered one and was amazed to find that out of twelve tests done, only one was normal. We got the child on IVs and corrected his hypovolemic (short of fluids in the vascular system) shock. Unfortunately, he went from that to a Gram negative shock (low blood pressure caused by substances released by bacteria that fail to gram stain). He was started on antibiotics and admitted to surgery since the source of all his problems seemed to be a bowel obstruction. The surgeons told me later he had responded well to the antibiotics, but none of them were willing to try to correct his problem because they thought it was just too dangerous. There was, at that time, a small proctology hospital in the city, and the child was transferred there where, after various enemas, they had had to go in with a proctoscope and physically remove the obstruction one spoonful at a time. After they got that cleared out, they found his bowel was about an inch thick, and there was a narrow point shown on the barium enema. They therefore went in and removed the narrow area and gave him a temporary colostomy. The narrow area represented an area of bowel without the normal nerves that cause it to contract. This condition is called Hirschsprung's Disease and is normally discovered shortly after birth. The mother had controlled it so well it didn't get the attention of the physicians until now. The child did well and eventually had his colostomy reconnected and didn't need enemas any more.

Sometimes we were presented with extremely difficult decisions. A young (fifteen-year-old) woman came complaining of vaginal bleeding after a miscarriage. During the exam, I asked what had happened and she said she'd felt a lot of pressure and passed two fetuses into the toilet. She said one of them cried. Of course, my ears really perked up at that. We immediately sent the police and an ambulance to the home where they found two premature infants dead in the toilet. On exam one of them had in fact breathed and then drowned. This information brought in detectives followed by the assistant DA and eventually a judge. Their initial thought was to charge the girl with murder, but they finally agreed she was so immature they wouldn't charge her. She simply didn't recognize that these were viable infants.

We were getting teenagers with some sort of overdose, which acted like an opiate. Finally, one day, one of them was brought in with a small paper bag of pink round pills. These were unlike any pill I was familiar with but looked to be commercial, so I sent them to our pharmacist. He said they looked vaguely familiar and after thinking a while went to a bottle of Darvon Compound and taking a capsule and opening it dumped out the powder inside, and out of the capsule there rolled my pink pill. After doing research we found that the Darvon chemically reacted with the aspirin in the compound so the company had placed the Darvon in a pill and the aspirin was there in powder form. The kids had apparently figured this out and were taking the Darvon pills out of the capsules in their parent's prescriptions, leaving the aspirin. They would then cook the Darvon and shoot it getting an opiate-like effect while their parents were taking aspirin only. Studies have since shown that the aspirin was probably the more effective of the two for pain.

An ambulance came in one day with a very large man who was bluish and panicking.

The story was that he'd collapsed while eating and was unable to breathe. We got him into an exam room, and I got the ambulance crew to help my people to hold him down while I put a laryngoscope into his mouth to look and see if I could see the obstruction. All I could see was a tiny piece of gristle coming out of his vocal cords. I used some special forceps designed to place breathing tubes in the trachea to grasp this piece and pulled gently, fearing it would break off. To my utter amazement, a complete slice of roast beef slid out of the trachea. It was rolled up like a scroll and neatly fitted the trachea. As soon as this piece was out, the patient began coughing and breathing. That was one of the more grateful patients I've had over the years. We let him rest for a while, and after a discussion about chewing his food, he was on his way none the worse for wear.

One evening we received a patient by ambulance who allegedly had hit a car head on at seventy miles per hour on his motorcycle, going through the wind shield of the car. He was, needless to say, severely injured, and one of the first things I noticed while working to stabilize him was he was paralyzed from the waist down. I assumed he had fractured his back or neck but X-rays failed to show any fractures. They did show the aorta was very wide and as we found later the deceleration had been so great his heart and aorta (the large artery coming out of the heart and going down to the body and legs) had been pulled forward. In doing so the small arteries that went back to his spinal cord had been torn off, leaving his spinal cord without a blood supply and therefore leaving him paralyzed. The surgeons rushed him off to surgery, but there was little hope with the technology we had then. Shortly after he was taken to surgery, the family arrived, including an elderly grandfather. They were sent to the surgery waiting room, and I heard later when the surgeon came to tell them the patient had died on the table, the grandfather had collapsed with a heart attack and had to be admitted to the coronary care unit.

Family disputes can frequently turn violent, but one of the more bizarre cases I've seen was a fight between a farmer and his hired hand. Both men involved were in love with the same lady even though all the participants were over age seventy. The farmer finally shot the hired man with a twelve-gauge shotgun from a distance of about ten feet. The hired man was brought in with a hole in his low abdomen about four inches in diameter. The x-rays were spectacular with dozens of BBs all over the low abdomen. The patient was taken immediately to surgery where he eventually died on the table. The surgeon later came back to the ER to look again at the x-rays. He said the top of the bladder was missing and the large and small bowel were hit as were some of the large vessels, but what he had come to check on was the pubic bone, which they had found at surgery seemed to be missing. When we looked for it on the x-rays there was no sign of it. Apparently the BBs had drawn our eyes such that none of us ever realized the bone was totally gone.

One day we had a thirteen-year-old female brought in confused and fighting, with a high temp. When I examined her, her neck was rigid as a board, which is a sign of irritation of the lining around the brain and spinal cord called the meninges. That, coupled with the fever, indicated meningitis until proven otherwise. We needed to get an IV in to give us a place to give medication. The young lady appeared to be physically in excellent shape, and I later learned she was a competitive swimmer. With several nurses holding her down, I got an IV into her anticubital fossa (the front of the elbow where there is a fairly consistent vein). I taped an arm board (a short padded board) across her elbow, but when we eased off, she snapped the board with ease. We managed to save the IV and with use of two boards taped together managed finally to protect her IV. I had not previously seen what confused people can do and how strong they can be.

Another problem arose when her mother told me she was allergic to penicillin, which would also preclude using ampicillin. Since the spinal tap revealed a gram negative diplococcal organism (a quick way to generalize types of bacteria), the penicillin group would have been the drugs of choice. We had just received the first of a new group of drugs called cephalosporins, which should work on these bugs but didn't appear to get into the normal brain. I decided that since other antibiotics didn't cross the normal meninges but did when the meninges were inflamed, our best bet was to try this new medication, and the attending, after talking with the pharmacy, agreed. Fortunately our guess was right, and the young lady turned the corner almost overnight. I was stuck with taking three days' worth of sulfa to prevent me from getting this nasty infection. There was enough meningitis in the area it seemed like I was on medication almost all year, but really I only had to take three or four courses.

Sometimes we'd get into conflict with local businesses. We had a large slide at an amusement park, which apparently had braces on the insides of the slide. The users were supposed to cross their arms across their chests while coming down but there were always some who didn't listen and put their hands down. This could result in a broken hand. The end of the slide also had a slight up angle and tended to throw people up into the air. I had one patient who came in with a fractured spinal process (those points you can see on the back) from being tossed in the air and landing on her back and another patient with a broken hand. Since this was clearly a design flaw, I contacted the company, who were totally uncooperative, so I contacted the Health Department and they sent an inspector out. After that we didn't see any more patients from that slide for several months. When another broken hand came in, they told us the slide people were most insistent they go to another ER rather than us. So much for problem solving.

We had a large manufacturer in the area who made a number of cleaning products and aerosols. They would have an accident every so often, and we'd get two or three patients by ambulance who were very upset, usually claiming they had difficulty breathing. I would have to call the company to find out what they had been exposed to since the patients never seemed to know. The company would always tell me that was a proprietary secret, but after considerable hassling, I would contact the plant physician who would swear me to secrecy and tell me what the substance was. It always turned out that the substance was harmless, but the employees didn't know it and had panicked.

My internship was called a rotating "o," which required that I have four months of Medicine and the rest could be divided as the hospital and I wished. I ended up with four months of Medicine, two months of Surgery, Ob-Gyn, and ER and one month of Pediatrics as well as one month of preceptorship. Interns were assigned a panel of GPs to whom we were responsible when they admitted patients. This meant we would do the history and physical and write the admitting orders, which would then have to be approved by the admitting physician.

One GP on my panel was one of my nightmares. This was a very well-regarded physician who was in his eighties and had become so senile that, after I worked for a year on his patients, he would still come to me and introduce himself as if we had never met. I guess nobody had the courage to tell him it was time to quit. At the time of writing this book, I have retired, and if what you are reading makes sense, then I guess I haven't reached that stage yet.

There were so many interns needing to take Medicine rotations they had to invent a special one for me consisting of Medicine ICU and CCU (intensive care unit and coronary care unit). This was a very good deal for me because I got to do a lot of hands-on procedures. My first ICU admit was an elderly black lady whose home had been fire-bombed and who had about 60 percent burns on her body. We had a burn unit as part of the ICU and got these patients referred to us. When I saw this lady in the ER, I could still smell the gasoline on her. No one knew why she had been attacked except she was black. She also turned out to have diabetes, and the internist who was assigned to admit her was so pessimistic about her chances he just told me to write whatever orders I wanted and he left. I decided that wasn't going to fly and began aggressive fluid therapy (now I was glad for the fluid therapy team training when I was a student). I worked on her all night, and in the morning I had her stabilized when the attending came in to make rounds. He was surprised to see her still there but went ahead and called the plastics-burn specialist to start trying to repair all the skin damage. We had a cream called Silvadeen, which had just been developed at the Brook Army Hospital for Vietnam wounded and started her with that. I was required to take her to whirlpool daily and remove the charred skin and blisters, which hurt her a lot even though we premedicated her with morphine. When she had healed enough, she had extensive skin grafting. Eventually she walked out of the hospital.

I had a second bad burn that month. The patient was a man in his mid-forties who had been on a hunting trip and was sleeping in a pickup camper when his gas lantern exploded. The only way out of the camper was through the back door. The lantern was, of course, between him and the door so he had to rush through the flames. As I recall he had about 35 percent burns, and though he had considerable pain, he survived.

Since I had the CCU as part of my responsibilities, I would get called at night if there was a cardiac arrest or life-threatening emergency. I had to cover every other night but could go home to sleep if things seemed quiet. Therefore I'd be sound asleep when the CCU nurses called a code blue, which means the patient has arrested or is about to arrest. I would bound out of bed and throw on my whites and run to the back door of the hospital. Usually by the time I got there, the nurses had the situation under control. I often would end up very light-headed as my adrenalin dropped, and I would have to lie down on an empty bed to prevent myself from fainting.

One evening one of the older attendings came in with a lady in her eighties who was a pediatrician in the upper peninsula of Michigan. I didn't know this attending, but he called me into the office and told me to go ahead and write some orders to keep her comfortable because he didn't think she would live until morning. When I looked at her ECG, it was apparent she had a posterior heart attack, and as is frequent with these, her heart was slowing to the point where it couldn't sustain her blood pressure. We did not yet have cardiac-pacing equipment, but I knew that atropine would at least temporarily block the vagus nerve, which was causing the problem, so I started to administer this drug with immediate response. We had to use the medication several times during the night, but by morning, much to the surprise of the attending, the lady was cheerfully taking breakfast and seemed stable.

As I recall, most, if not all, the patients in our CCU actually had heart attacks as opposed to today where the majority of patients in the chest pain unit do not have heart pain but some other source of chest pain such as esophagitis. We didn't have good laboratory tests such as the cardiac enzymes we use today, and cardiac cath was not a readily available diagnostic procedure. As a result we went by symptoms and the ECG, and since ECG changes were seldom from anything but the heart, we rarely admitted anything but heart attacks but missed a lot of heart problems, which would be picked up today. We also have interventions available today, which weren't available then, so missing a heart attack wasn't as consequential.

One day I received a code blue call from the ICU. When I arrived, I found a man in complete arrest. He was there to receive antibiotics for an infection of a heart valve, and another intern had just finished giving him an IV dose of penicillin. He resuscitated very quickly and without defibrillation, and we set out to find what had happened. The intern had gotten the IV lines confused and had injected the medication into the CVP (central venous pressure), a catheter run into the vena cava (the large vein, which returns blood to the heart) to measure pressures to determine if the heart is backing up. This line, since it is placed just above the inflow to the right atrium, allowed the medication to go directly to the heart without much dilution. Since the antibiotic was the potassium salt of penicillin, the potassium caused the heart to essentially spasm and stop. The hospital established a rule that only sodium penicillin could be pushed IV after that.

Pediatrics was a rotation with a mixed bag of things to do. One of our biggest jobs was to do pre-op histories and physicals on the "squints" who were scheduled for corrective surgery. I was initially put off by the word "squint" until I discovered it is an accepted diagnosis for cross eyes. These cases always came in Sunday afternoon for surgery on Mondays and there could be ten or more on the schedule. We got very fast at doing these especially since most of the kids were otherwise healthy.

We had one two-year-old brought in and admitted after getting into his mother's purse and taking a diet pill. These pills are strong stimulants, such as amphetamine, and are very dangerous in children. This baby was flying and we had to pad the crib to keep him from hurting himself. He ran around and around the crib while using his entire vocabulary, which consisted of "dada, mama, bye-bye, doggy" repeated over and over. After a few hours he finally settled down and was sent home the next morning. I realized that mother's purses are one of the most dangerous things children are around.

The pediatric rotation included responsibility for the neonatal unit, which was a source of frustration for me. There were no pediatric residents at our hospital and therefore only attendings to ask for help, and most of them were primarily involved with their offices, so we sometimes felt pretty much on our own. We had an anencephalic baby born in the hospital and sent to our unit. These babies are born without much of their brain and with their skull open. There was no chance for them to live, and we were told to just put them in the unit and wait for death. This one was still very much alive at the end of four days, so the attending cut off all water to the child and he finally died. I found that upsetting but I couldn't argue with the logic.

We were a large hospital so we got referrals from the smaller towns. One of these was a premature baby with respiratory distress syndrome (RDS). This is a breathing disorder of underdeveloped lungs. When I told the attending I knew very little about this disorder, he just looked at me with a very sad expression and said to do the best I could. Having laid this wonderful guidance on me, he went back to his office. The baby was working so hard to breathe he couldn't feed, so I called a surgical resident to help me do a cut down (cut down to a vein and insert a tube for IV fluid) and started to carefully balance fluids as well as I could. We didn't have micro blood gases, which we would use today, and I don't think we had a breathing machine for this size infant, so there was very little chance of saving the baby, who finally died. I would have felt much better if the attending had told me that not only did I know nothing about treating this disorder, neither did anyone else, which is why I could find nothing in the books either.

One of the diseases we would see fairly regularly was whooping cough. We rarely see it in children today but still see it in adults whose shots have worn off. At that time not all children were getting vaccinated, and we saw it as a kid's disease. You may have seen a snotty-nosed kid but you have seen nothing until you see whooping cough. These children made huge amounts of mucus and were very miserable. We did have one room designed for whooping cough and croup, which was completely tiled and could be turned into a steam room to aid in keeping the mucus runny so the child could clear it. The nurses hated that room because of what the steam did to their hair.

One of the procedures we were expected to know was the exchange transfusion. These were used to treat infants of Rh-mothers whose babies were Rh+. The Rh factor, if it crossed into the mother's blood, would stimulate an antibody response. The antibodies would get into the baby and attack his red blood cells. These babies were very sick, and their red blood cells were breaking down rapidly, so the treatment was to do a total blood replacement. This meant getting an IV in them and completely replacing their blood with Rh-blood, which wouldn't be attacked and wouldn't bother them either. Over time the antibodies would disappear and the child would do fine. Because of changes in the prevention of this disorder, I only did one exchange after internship and this disorder is pretty much a thing of the past. It can turn up in certain religious groups since the preventive is a blood-derived product, which some groups refuse.

That year I saw my first milk baby. This was one of a set of twins born to a poor family. The one twin progressed to solid food, but this one didn't like solids, and since it was cheaper anyway, the mother continued to feed this baby exclusively on breast milk. The child was now about eighteen months and was very lethargic and pale looking when brought in, especially when compared with his twin. Blood studies showed the child to be extremely anemic. Milk is not a complete food in that it lacks iron, and an exclusive diet will eventually result in anemia. When a baby is born, it has more red cells than needed because the oxygen levels in the uterus are low, but once it's breathing air, the levels are much higher, and the excess iron holds the infant for several months but is eventually used up. We got the mother to spend time with the dietician and started the baby on iron supplements, and he improved rapidly.

Ob-Gyn had only one resident so the intern got to do a lot more than on some of the other services. We had house staff cases from a small welfare clinic we ran on the hospital grounds, and the resident had to rotate to a facility for unwed mothers elsewhere as well. We were also expected to help the attendings with their cases, and that could be tricky. One day a patient came in in active labor, and the nurses had called her physician at his office to come in to deliver her. He was notorious for being late, and the patient was progressing rapidly, so I had them move her to the delivery room and call him again. When he still didn't show up, I decided to put in a nerve block called a pudendal to get her ready and save time. Usually these would take about three or four minutes to take effect, but just as I was removing the needle, in walked the attending. This man was known among the house staff as "the snake" because he'd seem nice and then strike like a snake. He asked what I'd done and I told him I'd put in a pudendal block. He walked to the table, grabbed a clamp, and put it on the patient's labia.

Fortunately for me she didn't feel it (fortunately for her as well), and he was impressed. I must have hit the nerve directly.

We had a pair of brothers (identical twins) who were both Ob-Gyns and practiced together. Their patients always wanted their own doctor to deliver them. They never really knew who had done their delivery, and the twins wouldn't tell them. The house staff could tell them apart after working with them for a while, but the patients never did. One day I got paged to the operating room stat (drop everything and run). When I arrived, I found one of the brothers doing a very fast scrub and rushing into the OR. I followed, and as I got there I found a very pale young woman with a distended abdomen, on the table being put to sleep. The second she was unconscious, he made a very fast incision and blood came gushing from the abdominal cavity. My job was to use suction and towels to clean up the blood so he could see to stop the bleeding. The story was that the young woman had been from out of town and had turned up in the office of one of our better GPs, complaining of being very early in pregnancy and having severe abdominal pain. She collapsed in his waiting room and he'd shipped her by ambulance while calling the Ob-Gyn attending to warn him so they'd brought her directly to the OR.

Once we were in the abdomen, I was able to remove the blood enough that the surgeon could see the source of the bleeding and get a clamp across it. We were then able to catch our breath and allow anesthesia to gain on her with blood and fluids. When you open an abdomen like that, the blood pressure usually drops suddenly because the blood in the abdomen had been holding back the bleeding because of the pressure of the distended abdomen. Once things were stabilized, we were able to go ahead and the remove the ovary where the pregnancy had implanted and repair the defect. Most ectopic pregnancies implant in the tube, but occasionally they'll get hung up on the ovary. As the fetus tries to grow, the blood vessels in the area grow to supply its needs, and when it finally ruptures (they usually do), the bleeding is rapid and the mother can die in a short period of time. This young woman was extremely lucky to walk out of the hospital even though she did lose an ovary and the pregnancy.

One of the attendings admitted a lady in labor who was undergoing her sixteenth pregnancy. She was a farm wife and her husband was with her. She'd delivered several of her babies at home but had decided to see an obstetrician for whatever reason. After we got her admitted and placed in a labor room, the attending went to the doctor's lounge to smoke a cigarette (most docs smoked in those days) and after finishing suggested we go check her again since he didn't think the labor would take long. When we entered the labor room we found her with the baby's head about to deliver and with her husband looking on with interest. Neither of them had called us or the nurse to let someone know what was happening. We went ahead and finished the delivery in the labor bed, and everybody was just fine. I still don't know why they bothered to come to the hospital.

The most anemic patient I've seen was admitted to Gyn, and I was the intern assigned to work her up. She complained that she'd had vaginal bleeding for months and was feeling tired and could hardly get through her day. When her blood work came back, her hematocrit came back at nine with the normal being above thirty-six, so she was running on about a quarter of the normal number of red cells. She felt much better after we transfused her and the attending started her on hormones to stop her bleeding. I wasn't convinced this was the answer because the lady was over seventy and hormones should no longer be a factor. She was discharged but I told her if the bleeding continued she needed to let her doctor know. Several days later the family called me to say she was still bleeding and they didn't trust their doctor and they didn't know what to do. I felt I was in a bad position because I was just an intern, so I went to the chief of Ob-Gyn and explained the situation. He had the family come in to the ER and he admitted the lady who was already fairly anemic again. A biopsy of the uterine lining showed uterine cancer and she subsequently underwent a hysterectomy. Hopefully she did well because I never heard about her after that.

We had another tricky legal issue turn up on Ob-Gyn. We were called by Medicine about a fifteen-year-old black girl in crisis. She turned out to be six weeks pregnant and had SC disease. SC is a blood disorder, which is composed of one sickle gene (largely found in blacks) and one hemoglobin C gene, which is also abnormal. The result is an abnormal red blood cell, which is very fragile. When these start breaking down, they cause severe abdominal pain and can even cause death. One of the things that will cause these to break down is pregnancy. In those days abortion could only be done on a court order and we had to go before a judge and swear that in our medical opinion this girl would die of her disease before she could deliver. We did this and got the court order, and she underwent the abortion. The night after the surgery, she again went into crisis, and I sat up all night pushing morphine for pain control and keeping her on oxygen. She survived. They had put an IUD in at the surgery and we also started her on birth control pills. We had discussed sterilizing her, but since she was so young, we felt there was a chance better treatment would be developed and she might be able to have children in the future.

As the year progressed we were beginning to think about specialties and we were asked if any of us were interested in general practice. I was one of three or four interns who indicated such an interest. There was a GP from upstate who had a small group with a small hospital, and this man had approached the hospital looking for a new partner. He invited us up to his hospital and showed us and our wives around a very nice facility, which was right next door to his equally modern office. He then took us to his home where we had dinner with him and one of his partners. During dinner he made a fatal error. He was quite an outdoorsman and talked of having to make his way to the hospital on his snowmobile in the winter because the snow was so heavy. He then told us laughingly about getting lost in a blizzard and ending up on the frozen river behind his house. We sort of looked at each other and that was the end of his chances of recruiting any of us. Many of us still felt uncomfortable with the level of training we had and it was scary thinking of going out and practicing right after internship.

Our surgical rotation was mostly memorable for the number of physicals we had to do pre-op. On Sunday when there was only one intern working, we might have fifteen or sixteen admissions for surgery the next day, and you had to do them all except when the resident was feeling charitable and gave you a hand. This usually meant working long into the evening, dictating, and writing orders. The dictating system was remarkable in that there was a typist on duty who could type nearly as fast as you could speak. After dictating, you had to write pre-op orders, and by the time you could do this, the dictation would be back, (they had one of those vacuum tube systems) so you could read and sign it.

One of the times I got into the OR was with a surgeon who was a notorious practical joker. We needed to drain a very large abscess in the fat of a very obese lady who had recently had an appendicitis and formed the abscess in the fat under the incision. The surgeon made a small skin incision and then worked his finger into the abscess. He told me to work my finger down along his and feel the size of the abscess. When I had, I looked up to see both the surgeon and the nurse on the other side of the patient grinning. He then told me to take my finger out, anticipating that the abscess, under pressure, would squirt all over me.

We had one surgeon who hated women. He was only about five feet tall, and you could tell where he was making rounds by the number of nurses you found crying at the nurses' stations. The problem was he was one of the best surgeons we had and was boarded in both general surgery and gynecological surgery. He was a retired military surgeon and expected everything to be done exactly as he wanted. I've seen him wash his hands, turn around with his hands out, expecting the nurse to drop a towel over them, chew out any nurse who failed to do so. The hospital refused to give him a scrub nurse when he did surgery because he upset the scrub nurses so badly, and they couldn't escape, so he had his personal scrub nurse who was as tough as he was and would walk out of the OR, if he got too nasty, until he came out and apologized. One night I was in the ER when we needed the surgeon on call, and it happened he was it, so I called him myself since he was always nice to the interns, rather than make the ward clerk call him as we usually would. His wife answered, and you could hear her yell, "A.J. get your a—out of bed. They need you at the hospital." Now I knew why he hated women. He arrived about twenty minutes later and started screaming at the nurses as he came through the door.

One of our favorite activities was to make "candy rounds," which consisted of going from nursing station to nursing station to see if a patient had given them candy, which was left out on the desk. Interns never got candy, but one time we had a big chocolate cake turn up in the intern's locker room marked as coming from the student nurses. The hospital had its own nursing school, which required the students to live in an attached dorm and do such things as undergo inspections in the morning, which determined whether or not they got to go out that weekend. The student nurses were not wildly in love with the interns since they were the only ones lower on the pecking order, so we were a bit suspicious of this cake. Some of the interns relabeled the cake to the administration from the student nurses and took it to the administrative office. They were too trusting and some of them ate this cake. It turned out the chocolate frosting was made out of Ex-Lax, and several administrators were out the next day with the "stomach flu."

My three months of regular Medicine rotation was largely spent doing workups and writing orders on patients with heart, liver, and blood diseases. We also saw a fair amount of cancer and congestive heart failure. One day I was called to work up a patient with the diagnosis of "dropsy" sent in by the very elderly attending on my GP panel. Dropsy is a very old term for some form of fluid retention. It became readily apparent that the lady had severe ascites, which is fluid collecting in the abdomen. She had so much fluid she had trouble moving her diaphragms against the pressure. After doing the history and physical, I decided to drain some of the fluid off so she would be more comfortable. This is called a paracentesis and is really a very simple procedure of placing a small tube in the abdominal cavity and draining the fluid slowly, relieving the pressure, which also served a useful purpose of giving us material to make the diagnosis. The pathology department was able to find cells of ovarian cancer in the fluid. After that we just did what we could to make the lady comfortable until she expired since it was so widespread and there was no treatment at that time.

As luck would have it, one of my patients on Medicine was one of the staff gynecologists. He'd been on vacation in the Caribbean and done the classic cartoon maneuver of stepping back one more step while taking a picture and falling over a cliff. He'd landed in a tree and one of the limbs had punctured his abdomen and lacerated his liver. He'd been operated on there, and by the time he was ready to come home, he was turning jaundiced. It was not clear whether this was something to do with the injury or whether he'd gotten hepatitis from all the blood transfusions he'd received. He was admitted for observation and testing and placed on a high protein diet. He was virtually addicted to his daily two or three martinis and was very upset that we told he couldn't drink. One day, the resident and I were making rounds on him when we smelled something funny. He had a large bouquet of flowers from which this odor of junipers was coming. He'd somehow convinced his friends to replace the water in the vase with gin, which we took away. I never understood whether he'd been a gynecologist for so long he no longer understood liver failure could kill you or whether he just didn't care.

We had one admission of a local college president who was having such a sore throat he couldn't swallow liquids. When examined, he had huge pus-covered tonsils and large lymph nodes in his neck. Lab tests confirmed he'd contracted infectious mononucleosis probably from one of the college students he was in contact with. He improved in a few days of IV fluids, but the case impressed me with how severe this disease can get.

I had one month of preceptorship, which consisted of two weeks with a country GP and two more weeks with a city GP. I was given this since I had expressed an interest in general practice. The country GP was the only doctor in a small town nearby and had been there for many years. He had gone there right out of internship, which was common in those days and had had to learn many things out of a book. He described doing a lumbar puncture with a book on a stand next to him because he'd never done one in training. This man was in his seventies, and I was in my twenties and he could work me into the ground. His office was open six days a week, and he had night hours Tuesday and Thursday. When we broke for lunch or dinner, he would make several house calls before going home and gulping down a meal.

He tried to keep up to date, but since he worked such hours, it was really difficult. He had one young lady come with a typical "butterfly rash" and I wondered if she might have Lupus. He was unfamiliar with the syndrome, but he had a pretty up-to-date library in the basement of his office, and we were able to look it up and confirm the diagnosis.

The urban GP worked in an office of three GPs. He and one partner saw the majority of the patients and were very familiar with the patients. The third man was older and interested in psychiatric cases.

My preceptor told me he and the other GP were very happy to have their older colleague see these cases, so they could concentrate more on medical cases.

As I said, this man knew his patients very well. We were called to the ER for a ten- or eleven-year-old boy who was his patient and probably had a fracture. When we arrived, the films were already out and confirmed a fracture of his radius and ulna known as a Colles' fracture. The freckle-faced tough-looking redhead sitting there told us he'd fallen on a rock. My preceptor told me to watch this kid as he set the fracture. He asked the boy if he wanted anesthesia, and he said no, so my preceptor went ahead and set the fracture without any. The kid just sat there and looked on interestedly as if he felt nothing. The preceptor told me later the kid had had several fractures and never needed anesthesia.

During the internship, decisions had to be made regarding the armed forces. At that time, the service was nearly universal for physicians because the Vietnam conflict was going strong. You really had two choices. You could wait to be drafted or you could volunteer. I felt that volunteering was more sensible and joined the air force reserve. There was also a plan called the Berry Plan, which allowed you to finish residency before going on active duty. If you were accepted for that, you were guaranteed to finish your residency and to be allowed to practice your specialty when on active duty. I was interested in the new specialty being developed called Family Practice and applied for the Berry Plan in that specialty and was accepted.

As the internship was nearing its end, I started looking for residencies. As I mentioned earlier, I was interested in Family Practice, which was a new specialty that had not received approval yet, so it was a bit of a gamble. I had investigated several developing residencies and settled for one that was an established GP residency. The GP residency was not needed to become a GP, but several residencies, especially in California, had been established. The one I finally settled on was run by one of the physicians who was very involved in developing Family Practice as a specialty, and I thought it likely his residency would be accredited early, which proved to be the case.

I applied and was startled to get a phone call from the director himself one day to tell me if I wanted to come, I was accepted. I agreed and so was set to move back to the West Coast.

The move back was the move from hell. We had rented the largest U-Haul trailer made and it was loaded full. We were going to pull it with our little Buick Skylark. The day we started out was also the first day of a heat wave, and our car was running hot. We weren't out of the state when I noticed a number of cars pulled over and changing tires. I realized there were a number of small metal objects on the road, and these were causing flats. I stopped to check and found one of the tires on the trailer hissing as it slowly went down. There was a sign for U-Haul at a filling station off the highway, and I pulled in there to get the tire fixed. The men working there didn't seem to be the sharpest knives in the drawer, but they agreed to fix the tire. Since we were running hot, I asked if they could also take out the thermostat to allow a little more cooling. They agreed, and I stationed myself by the engine compartment to make sure the fellow doing that knew what he was doing. He was doing fine, but I realized the car seemed to be at a funny angle, and when I looked, I found the fellow working on the tire had put a jack under the back of the trailer and put the entire trailer weight on the rear of our car which was now on the ground. I got that corrected; after they finished their jobs, we got on our way.

There was a heat wave across the country, and we traveled right in the middle of it. By the time we got to Oklahoma, we were traveling at night and still could only go a few miles before the engine overheated and we had to stop to let it cool. I called U-Haul to see if we could rent a pickup to pull the trailer. They had one in Norman, Oklahoma, which was a little out of our way, but we reserved it anyway. Driving at night, we got to Norman a little after dawn and had to sit and wait for U-Haul to open.

We finally got the trailer transferred to the pickup, and I drove the pickup while Sue drove our car. I had not thought what it would be like driving an empty pickup pulling a very heavy trailer, but it's somewhat akin to riding a bronco. Every time I hit a bump the heavy trailer would jerk the pickup and slam it down into the road, but at least nothing was overheating.

We knew the desert crossing was going to be tough with the heat continuing, so we made confirmed reservations at a motel in Needles and planned on arriving there very early in the morning and sleeping the day away. We were still traveling at night, and when we reached Flagstaff, Sue started flashing her lights at me. I found a place to pull the truck and trailer over and went back to see what the problem was now. She said the car was making funny noises, and after driving around the block, I had to agree so we waited several hours until a filling station opened at 7:00 a.m. The mechanic (they had mechanics in filling stations in those days) put the car on the lift and found the sound was coming from the rear axle bearings. He took the axle out and said several of the bearings looked like they'd been flattened by a heavy weight. I immediately thought of our genius tire changer.

We had to wait another hour until a machine shop opened to turn our axle and then it had to be reinstalled with new bearings. We finally left Flagstaff and started into the desert about ten in the morning when we'd planned on arriving at Needles. Because we had confirmed reservations, we were going to be charged for the room regardless of whether we got there or not. So we decided to go on.

The desert really heated up and I guessed it was around 120° F when the truck began overheating. I found that by turning the heater on in the truck, I got just enough additional cooling that the engine wouldn't overheat. I was guessing the temp in the cab was about 140° F even with all the windows open. We made it to Needles before I collapsed, and I had several Cokes with ice before I recovered.

We arrived in Los Angles on the Fourth of July and had to take the freeway to where my residency was located. The freeway had signs saying trailers must stay in the right-hand lane and I didn't know if they were referring to small trailers or not, so I decided I'd better try to stay in that lane. The problem began when they added lanes to the freeway and I discovered there was no right-hand mirror on the truck. I couldn't see the lane because of the trailer, so I just turned on my turn blinker for a long time, assuming Sue would move over to give me room. She, unfortunately, didn't read my mind. When I finally pulled off because I was a nervous wreck and wanted to find an alternate route, she asked me if I knew I'd nearly driven several cars off the road.

Residency

When we got to our new home, we found an apartment, which had all the charm of a motel room, but it was a month to month so we could go out looking for something better, eventually finding a house, which was memorable for a night-blooming jasmine outside the bedroom window and a roll-around dishwasher (our first).

The hospital was stucco with a red tile roof in the Southern California style. It sat in a complex of buildings that included the psychiatric inpatient unit, the jail hospital unit, the infectious disease unit as well as other county buildings such as the welfare office and the coroner's office.

There were a total of five residents in my class. Originally there were supposed to be six, but one fellow used his residency contract to get out of the draft and then disappeared. I guess he hadn't figured on our education director having worked his way through medical school as a bill collector. He tracked the fellow down, and the county sued him for the cost of hiring an additional physician to work the clinics.

We received the usual welcome speech from the director and then were given a tour of the hospital by the director of Ob-Gyn. He was younger than most of the department heads and was one of the few who weren't "dollar a year" men. These were private physicians who were paid one dollar a year, so they were technically employed by the hospital thus covered by the malpractice insurance. There was a two-tiered system with a junior attending and a senior attending. The junior attendings were mostly GPs who had graduated from our program, and the senior attendings were conventional specialists. There were six senior residents as well, including the chief resident.

As we were walking around the building, there was an "any resident to OB stat" page over the loud speaker. We all ran up the one flight to the fourth floor OB department where the nurse directed us to the labor room. There we found a lady with a baby in a breech position delivered out to the umbilicus. I had never delivered a breech but knew the theory and knew that since the cord was compressed at that point, the baby needed to be delivered as quickly as possible. I was expecting the OB chief to step in, but he and all the other residents just stood there staring, so I stepped up and finished the delivery, which was my first breech delivery.

Once we were oriented, we received our assignments for the year, which were in one- or two-month rotations on all the major specialties with time in outpatient clinics as well. You were primary call every eleventh night and secondary call at the same interval. Primary call stayed in the hospital all night and worked in the ER but was also responsible for the inpatient units including OB, after the secondary doctor call went home at ten or eleven. You tried very hard not to call the secondary guy back in because you didn't want him to call you back when he was primary. You did have a place to sleep, but it was in an empty ward in the back of the hospital and you rarely got to use it. That part of the hospital had been closed for some time and was pretty creepy, so it was no big loss. The residents on surgery were on call every other night because if surgery was needed, the primary call couldn't be tied up that long.

When a patient came in at night and looked like he needed admission, the ER doc would write a note and admitting orders, and the resident to whom the patient was admitted would complete the work-up in the morning. One such patient was admitted to my service with pneumonia. When I came in in the morning, I found an elderly chronic alcoholic who was very confused and running a fever. He had had multiple admissions in the past but had not been confused. Examination showed not only the expected breath sounds of pneumonia, but also he had a very stiff neck. I did a lumbar puncture, which confirmed bacterial meningitis, and later the cultures showed pneumococcus. I transferred him out to the infectious disease ward, which was in a separate building behind the main hospital and started him on high doses of IV antibiotics. His mental faculties did not improve over the next several days, either because the meningitis wasn't responding, because of the hypoxia (low oxygen level) caused by his pneumonia, or because the chronic alcoholism had finally finished off his brain. Therefore, I was forced to re-tap his spinal fluid to see how much response we were getting. The infectious disease unit was run by an older maidenly nurse who had to hold the patient while I did his tap because motion with a needle in the spinal canal is dangerous. As I was putting the needle in, I heard the nurse saying, "Stop that, stop that, you dirty old man." I looked up to see the patient had gotten a hand loose and was feeling under her skirts. I decided he wasn't as confused as I had thought. Barely able to keep from laughing, I managed to finish the exam and sent the specimen to the lab.

The patient eventually recovered, but his brain never worked as well as it should have, and we discharged him to a long-term care nursing home out in the country beyond walking distance of a bar. At least walking distance for him.

Another alcoholic contributed to one of my rare coups on Medicine. This was a lady in her mid-forties who was admitted with liver failure. She was obviously jaundiced and her mentation wasn't so great, but she was able to tell me she had a problem with alcohol, although she'd been able to hold down her regular job as a hairdresser until she fell ill a couple days earlier. By the morning after admission her kidneys shut down, and she went into hepato-renal failure, which was just about a death sentence in those days. I felt this was progressing way too fast for our usual alcoholic, and also she'd never even been bad enough to be admitted in the past. Alcoholics could present with this syndrome but usually only after numerous admissions for their liver problems, so I put her on the list for grand rounds. Grand rounds were held weekly, and all the residents on Medicine as well as the chief of Medicine and the residency director went to look at the difficult or unusual cases on the ward. This particular day the chief pathologist came with us as well. No one could explain why this patient was fading so quickly, but the pathologist said she looked like the tourists he'd seen as a boy. He'd grown up in the Middle East near the Dead Sea. He said the tourists would swim in the sea and occasionally one would swallow a mouthful. The salts in the sea would kill them. I asked what salts were involved since sodium chloride (table salt) in small quantities obviously wouldn't do this, and he told me they were bromates and perchlorates. Since I had no other leads, I went to the hospital library and got a chemistry book that listed the substances. I learned that bromates were used in permanent wave solution neutralizer. Since the patient used these every day, in her job as a hairdresser, I thought I'd found my culprit. Our lab couldn't test for bromates but they could test for bromides into which the body would convert a small amount of the bromates. The results showed much more bromide than expected, confirming my suspicion. About this time the patient died, and the coroner wanted the cause of death. I told him my suspicions and suggested his investigator go to her hairdressing cubicle and see if there weren't two bottles labeled as permanent wave solution neutralizer. My suspicion was that she drank between customers and had taken a slug from the wrong bottle. The investigator found two such bottles, one of which contained white wine.

Since we were a county hospital in Southern California, many of our patients were Mexican agriculture workers, many of whom did not speak English. We had interpreters and we also learned a little Spanish, but since many of the patients spoke a form of Spanish referred to as border Spanish, they frequently didn't know any anatomical terms nor did they have any medical terms. Our interpreters would substitute four letter words where they could, but it still was a major problem. One time I was seeing a child in the clinic who was about fourteen months old and had severe head trauma. X-rays showed the child's head was shattered like an egg shell. Since neither the mother nor her girlfriend spoke English, I sent for an interpreter because I was going to have to explain the child abuse laws to them. While we were waiting, the mother and her friend were discussing what story they were going to tell me. They didn't realize I spoke enough Spanish to know what they were doing. The story they gave was that the child had been sitting on the floor and had fallen over, striking his head. This, of course, was nowhere near enough trauma to cause the damage we were seeing. When the interpreter arrived, I explained I was admitting the baby for observation, although so far the exam showed no neurological damage. Once the baby was admitted, we called a judge we had on twenty-four-hour call, and he took custody of the child and turned it over to us. We also called the police who came out and arrested the mother. At that point she told us the real story. She'd had the baby in her arms when she stumbled, and the child's head hit the stub of a pipe sticking out of the wall in the picker's hut they lived in. She wasn't married to the father and was afraid he'd throw her out if he learned she was at fault. She was also afraid she'd be deported if the authorities were involved because she was here illegally. Had she given me the true story in the first place, the trauma would have matched the pathology, and I would not have had to bring in the police. As it was, she was transferred to Los Angeles County where they had a Spanish-speaking lie detector technician and her second story was confirmed. I never heard if immigration was informed. The baby did fine.

I came in one morning to find a patient had been admitted to me during the night with the story that he had been feeling normal, although his wife noted he was drinking over a gallon of iced tea a day. She decided this was not good for him, so she cut him off. Over the next day or two, he became increasingly somnolent and confused. For some reason the resident in the ER the night before had not done the usual orders stat, so no results were back, but since he had a catheter in place I went to check his output and found a few drops of urine, which was thick as syrup. When I had the lab move his lab up to stat I got back a blood sugar about eight to ten times normal at one gram. I moved him to the ICU and started fluid replacement and tiny amounts of insulin. If people in diabetic coma are corrected too quickly, they will have problems with too much fluid being sucked into their central nervous system and can die. This man was staving off coma by drinking large amounts of iced tea and peeing out large amounts of sugar until his wife decided to stop his drinking. He recovered nicely and probably was controlled on pills alone since he never had ketoacidosis like an insulin-dependent diabetic would.

One of our rotations was anesthesia, which is an interesting field. Anesthesia has been described as 90 percent boredom and 10 percent panic. There are two periods when the panic can occur, generally speaking; these are the induction (starting anesthesia) and waking the patient. There's always concern at those times, but much of the rest of the time is spent monitoring the patient's vital signs and sometimes doing things to help the surgeon.

We had one surgeon who was known as a screamer. He was a thoracic and vascular surgeon, and he not only worked on county patients, but he also brought his private patients to the county hospital so he could get resident coverage, which they didn't have at the private hospital in town. He really believed in the residents, and he really believed in his sleep so it all worked out.

One day I was giving anesthesia for him, and suddenly the heart monitor went crazy. The pattern didn't look like anything that would be coming from the patient, so I looked at the equipment and found the surgeon was standing on the line from the patient to my monitor. Since this surgeon was in the midst of a tricky job, I simply inflated the BP cuff far enough that I could hear the pulse and monitored that way until the surgeon glanced up and saw the monitor and started screaming that I wasn't watching his patient. I calmly explained the patient was fine and could he move his foot off the cord. He became very sheepish and apologized.

The surgical rotation was challenging. The residency director had been a GP surgeon for many years and was still the man the specialty surgeons would call when they were in trouble in the OR. Since we were in the West where there were a lot of small towns without access to large hospitals and standard specialists, the boss thought the residents should learn as much surgery as possible. Therefore, since we were a county hospital, all patients except the attendings' private ones were the resident's patients, and the boss felt if you could do the surgery you should. The attending was always there, and at any point you could ask him to take over.

One evening I was making rounds on the surgical floor, and a patient I had scheduled for a gallbladder surgery in the morning called to me as I walked past and told me she could feel a tearing sensation; she thought her gallbladder had ruptured. Being a resident, I thought I knew better and reassured her and got her a bigger dose of pain medication. The next morning she had a rigid abdomen, and we moved her to the top of the surgical schedule. We found her abdomen full of small gallstones, and to this day I can remember the boss with a large serving spoon they got from somewhere spooning gallstones out of the patient's abdomen. I had forgotten one of the primary rules to always listen to the patient. The lady recovered eventually, but it took longer than it should and she had more discomfort than was necessary.

We had a scrub nurse in surgery who probably taught the residents more about surgery than most of the attendings. She was a large Mexican lady and had been working in surgery and our orthopedic clinic for many years. If you weren't sure what to do next, you had only to hold out your hand and she would put the correct instrument in it, and you'd better figure out what to do with it. If you rejected her instrument, you'd never get another chance in that surgery. Likewise in the ortho clinic where we saw orthopedic patients following surgery as well as patients who generally had orthopedic complaints, she wouldn't tell you what you should do, but if you asked, she would say, "Dr. So and so would do this or that." She'd almost always be right. Nurses like this have saved me from myself many times.

We had one of the first fiber optic laparoscopes in the United States, our OB director having been flown to Chicago to receive instruction in its use. I had used it a number of times to do tubal ligations, which was one of the few uses we had in those days (it's used for many procedures in general surgery today). A friend of mine was a Public Health nurse, and she and her husband had decided they had enough children, so she came to me specifically to see if I'd do a laparoscopic tubal for her. I arranged it in surgery and we did the procedure. I noted during the surgery that it took more power to burn the tubes than usual, and when we removed the drapes we found out why. The insulation, which was only a painted coating, had been scratched when the scope was cleaned, allowing the scope to short out into the abdominal wall causing a burn there as well as at the tubes. Fortunately I had used a "Z" track technique when I put the instrument channel in and therefore the layers slid back over each other so the burn did not go straight through. We kept the patient overnight to be sure nothing else had happened, and she went home reasonably happy. When I saw her the next day for a dressing change she told me when she got home the phone was ringing and it was a lawyer who told her he'd heard what happened and that she had a very good case to sue the county. She refused, but the information clued us into the fact that he had a mole in the OR who tipped him off when something went wrong. We later caught the aide involved and fired him. My patient healed with minimal scarring and was happy with her choice in spite of everything.

Lawyers are a constant problem in medicine, sometimes for good but often not. I had one evening in the ER when the local police called me about a prisoner who had swallowed a large amount of heroin when he was arrested. As was common the heroin was contained in a number of condoms and the police asked if this could hurt him. I explained even balloons intended for use in the gut sometimes broke and that there was certainly a possibility these would as well. Since heroin is variably absorbed from the gut, the amount described could indeed kill him. They brought the prisoner in, and since he was in custody, they gave consent to empty his stomach. He refused to take the Ipecac we would normally use, so we used a substance called Apomorphine, which is given intramuscularly. In about five minutes he vomited up a quantity of condoms or balloons, which the police confiscated. I thought no more about it until some weeks later I got a call from an assistant DA telling me I was going to be subpoenaed on the case.

Later in court I found a person I barely recognized. The filthy, unwashed drug dealer I had seen in the ER had gotten a haircut and was clean and wearing a suit. I was called to the witness stand, but instead of the defendant's lawyer asking me questions, the judge asked all the questions in a most hostile way. It seemed the defense lawyer was claiming the medication constituted an illegal search of the patient's stomach and was not medically indicated. The ADA (assistant district attorney) tried to object but the judge just ignored him. After court the judge said I was without integrity and that it was indeed an illegal search and dismissed the case. The local paper picked up the story, and because of previous friction between them and the hospital, the article was very hostile. Associated Press also picked up the story, and the headline in the *LA Times* was "Judge Knocks Medico for Saving Life," which I thought was a bit more reasonable. The local medical society was willing to sue the judge since some of his remarks were made off the bench, but the judicial review by one of the members of the State Supreme Court resulted in the judge being given a reprimand and removed from any further criminal cases. The ADA told me later that not only had the "search" of the stomach been decided previously by the courts as not a search but medical treatment, but also this particular judge had had political ambitions and thought he was setting precedence.

I inherited a patient when we changed rotations and I went back to Medicine. This was a young Mexican field worker who was coughing up large amounts of blood daily from a lung problem. He had been tentatively diagnosed with an extremely rare lung disorder, which acted this way and was always fatal. It was getting harder and harder to get a blood match for him since he was requiring a unit daily to keep up with the loss. When you use so much blood, the patient gradually develops antibodies to the lesser antigens in blood, and it gets very hard to find a match. I was unhappy with the diagnosis since the disorder he had been diagnosed with always occurred in both lungs, and this appeared to be only in the right. Since it was apparent we were not going to be able to continue the transfusions, I talked with the chest surgeon about removing the bleeding lung since he could get along with one lung and he was going to die as things were going. The surgeon reluctantly agreed and took him to surgery. There he found a large abscess in that lung so he drained it and took samples for culture and biopsied the wall. Pathology found nothing in the abscess fluid, but the wall was full of a parasite called amoeba. This organism normally infests the bowel but sometimes gets into the liver and then can cross the diaphragm and form abscesses in the right lung. When we looked, we found several small abscesses in the liver, which had not been apparent. When he was started on the appropriate medications, he showed remarkable response and recovered rapidly. I saw this patient months later, and he had gone from a pale, skinny, sick young man to a healthy, muscular young man who was back in the field working and getting on with his life.

I also had a patient who was admitted with congestive heart failure and on admission was found to have early renal failure. She was a black lady who had a history of arthritic pain as well, and in spite of somewhat limited testing being available in those days, I was able to diagnose her as having Systemic Lupus Erythematosis, which in those days was usually considered a terminal illness. She eventually succumbed to her illness in spite of steroids, as did most patients at that time because one of the required criteria then was to have renal involvement before you could make the diagnosis. Today with better testing we know that much of lupus consists of primarily arthritis and does not always go on to the full-blown picture she had.

One night when I was covering the emergency I was called to the floor because a patient who was in restraints because he was going through DTs and was belligerent. He had gotten an arm loose and the nurses were afraid to get too close. When I arrived, I found a 250-pound man with one arm loose and swinging at anyone who came close. I managed to grab his free arm and was holding it down when I looked up and saw a giant fist coming down. I had not realized he'd been working the other hand loose as well. I managed to hit the floor and avoid being cold cocked, and three nurses finally got enough courage up to grab his other arm and apply leather restraints.

Like all ERs we had our regulars. One, I'll call Eddy, was a chronic alcoholic who hated to go to jail. Eddy had worked out that the police didn't want sick people in the jail, so every time he was arrested for being "drunk in public," Eddy would have a "seizure," and since seizures in chronic alcoholics weren't uncommon and there would be less paperwork, the cops would load him in an ambulance and ship him to the ER. When he arrived in the ER, I'd ask him how he was and he'd stop jerking around on the stretcher long enough to look at me and say, "It's really bad this time, Doc" and then resume his "seizure." One time a new ambulance crew had called ahead to tell us they were bringing in a patient in status epilepticus (unremitting seizures, which can be life threatening). When they arrived, my staff and I were waiting by the door, but to the amazement of the ambulance attendants, when we saw it was Eddy, we just went back to our other patients and left them standing there. One of the other residents had gotten tired of Eddy tying up the ER and always claiming upon leaving that we had stolen his wallet with $400 in it, so he pointed out Eddy never had a lumbar puncture with all these seizures. (A lumbar puncture consists of introducing a needle into the spinal column and collecting fluid for analysis. This would be an appropriate test for recurrent seizures). Since Eddy had absolutely no idea what this test was, he agreed to it. After prepping his back so there would be no infection, the resident poked him in the back with a needle several times causing Eddy to jump up cussing, make his usual accusations and leave. After that we had no trouble getting Eddy to go by simply reminding him that we never completed the test and needed to try again. Sometimes you have to out manipulate the manipulators.

One night the police brought in two little boys who had drunk much of a jug of wine. The officers said they became suspicious something was amiss when the boys pelted their patrol car with eggs as they drove by. When they caught them, they found these two-seven year-olds had stolen a jug of wine from a convenience store in the barrio and had drunk most of it. One of them passed out right after arriving, and I went ahead and put a tube in his stomach and got back about a quart of wine. Fortunately I ordered the standard battery of tests we did on unconscious patients, thinking there might be more than met the eye. I started an IV and put him in the ICU to be carefully watched. A short time later I got two calls at the same time. The ICU nurse called to say he was convulsing, and the lab called to say his blood sugar was 17. We pushed glucose on him and he immediately improved. I was unaware that since alcohol bypasses the glucose cycle and the brain can only use glucose, patients, especially children, can become severely hypoglycemic to the point of convulsions or causing brain damage.

Southern California has many motorcycle gangs and two of them caused one of the more memorable evenings in the ER. The Satan's Saints had a clubhouse in town, which was basically a bar where they hung out. The Hessians had had a motorcycle stolen and suspected the Saints of having stolen it. They showed up at the bar one Saturday afternoon, and the resulting war was fought with pool cues and motorcycle drive chains, which many of them would wear as belts. This resulted in numerous head injuries. The first two ambulances to arrive in my ER had managed to stuff in thirteen head injuries between them. I ended up calling for help from a couple of residents who were at home and even the radiologist came in. In those days we didn't have CT scans but did take X-rays of serious head injuries. We found two depressed skull fractures (the bone was broken and pushed down into the brain), so we had to call in the neurosurgery team to operate on those. The rest of the injuries were largely scalp and other lacerations. In order to get a clean field we normally would cut the hair in the area of the laceration and then sew it together. One big guy (about 6'5" and over 300 lbs.) sat straight up on his gurney and proclaimed, "Nobody cuts my hair." We all agreed we wouldn't think of doing such a thing. He was brought back from the jail because of continued bleeding the next day and a large scalp laceration was found hidden in the long, dirty hair.

The cops simply backed a Paddy Wagon up to the ER door and loaded the fighters in as fast as we could sew them up. One of the cops who had been on the scene told me they had arrived and could see what was happening and simply waited outside until things got quiet before going in, not wanting to get any officers injured. He claimed there was so much blood on the floor it was difficult to walk in there.

Walking back and forth to X-ray felt like walking by a Van-de-Graf generator with one gang's supporters on one side of the hall and the others on the other side; you could feel the sparks jumping back and forth. I heard one gang leader talking about bringing their other clubs in California (1,400 members) to finish the fight. I asked him if they could take the fight to Los Angeles County where they had bigger ERs, and he said they'd try since we had been so nice to them.

One of the gang members got a scalp infection in his wound, and we had to see him a number of times to treat it and drain it. He worked as a commercial fisherman and asked if one of the other residents and I would like to go fishing in return for our care. He arranged for us to go on a party boat he had worked on, and we caught a number of calico bass. He also later brought his girlfriend in to see me. She danced at a local topless bar and had a moderately severe case of gonorrhea.

In those days we used a great deal of balanced traction. This is the setup where pins are put into a broken bone and attached to weight to pull the bone straight. One night, while I was on the ER and the only doc in the hospital, I was called by the nurse in Orthopedics that they had a patient in traction who needed his Foley catheter changed. This catheter is held in the bladder by a small balloon and must be changed regularly to avoid infection. The nurses were unable to get the balloon to deflate and didn't know what to do. I went to the Ortho floor and found a scraggly motorcycle club member who had a Foley in place. He was covered with tattoos including one on the shaft of the penis, which said, "Hot Dog." I couldn't get the balloon to deflate either so I cut the side arm (where the inflation channel is) hoping it would deflate. It didn't but I was able to thread a blunt needle into the inflation channel and found I could put water in but it wouldn't come back. I reasoned the balloon was only so large so I just kept putting water in until the balloon popped resulting in an audible bang. The patient thought he'd lost everything and jumped straight up knocking weights every which way. The Foley came out easily after that. The next day the nurses told me the patient had requested I not see him, and I certainly was upset about that.

We had another episode that filled the hallway outside of the ER. This time it stemmed from a wedding reception where, among other things, they had commercially made jerky. Within two hours of eating this, the guests developed severe abdominal pain and explosive diarrhea. About twenty of these people hit us at once. Since our restroom space was limited, the nurses ended up distributing bedpans to the people in the hall, which became rather odiferous.

Naturally the Health Department got involved and went to the factory where the jerky was made. They found a Mexican national they had deported previously who was known to be a Salmonella carrier. The man had simply re-crossed the border and went back to work in meat processing without getting treatment for his carrier state. The company paid for their failure to follow the law by having to recall beef jerky, which had been distributed all up and down the West Coast.

One night I had a man brought in with a knife cut from ear to ear and deep enough to reach the muscle but not the major vessels. He told me he and his girlfriend had been in a fight and she had cut him. About that time a woman with several girlfriends walked in to get her black eyes checked out. We had a hard time finding her chart and when we did we found it had five or six different last names each crossed out and replaced with a new one.

I got her out as quickly as possible not wanting to get caught in a renewal of their fight as had an intern in the town where I had interned. He'd just started to examine a woman brought in with a gunshot wound from a fight with her husband when the husband showed up to finish her, and in the process killed the intern.

When I got back to the man with the knife wound, I advised him we could call the police if he wished, but he told me he really loved that woman, especially since she put up such a good fight. I just shut up and did a three-layer closure that took most of the night.

One day a small child in the waiting room of the ER suddenly began to choke and started to turn blue. The receptionist screamed for help, and the nurse and I went to the waiting room, and after turning the child upside down and a little back pounding, he coughed up a peanut. When we asked the mother where he got a peanut, she admitted to buying it from a vending machine in the lobby. We had the company remove peanuts and other small objects that could be inhaled in the future.

We had another child who came in with a persistent cough for the past couple days. His breath sounds had some wheezing to them so I got an x-ray of his chest and found a crucifix hanging in his epiglottis by its crossbars. We had to give him a couple breaths of nitrous oxide so we could remove it without creating panic.

In Southern California it gets pretty dry in the summer to the point of huge fires developing. Our area had several parks backed up to the dry hills, and these had to be watered to keep the grass green. The presence of water drew wildlife down from the dry hills to drink. One of the critters they drew was rattlesnakes. There were public service announcements warning people of this and suggesting if they did get bitten, they should kill the snake and bring it in to be identified because there are a number of snakes that will act somewhat like rattlers down to and including shaking their tails in dead leaves making a rattle like sound.

At that time there was some controversy about treatment and one study where they'd allowed snakes to bite dogs and then excised (cut out) the fang marks had found most of the venom could be removed if the excision was done in half an hour(not an experiment that could be done today). I had one child brought in with a bite on his leg that certainly could have been a rattler but they brought in no snake. It had just happened so I went ahead and excised the fang marks and underlying tissue down to the muscle. We then observed the child for several hours, and he never developed any swelling or other symptoms of the bite. I'll never know whether the bite was from a rattler and we got most of the venom or whether the snake had no venom but regardless the child went home with only a small scar.

Another patient came in with a snake bite, and I asked him if he'd killed the snake and brought it in and he said he had. He proceeded to dump the contents of a gunnysack on the ER floor and out came a very angry five-foot Diamond Back Rattler, which proceeded to scoot down the length of the ER with screaming patients and nurses running every which way. I finally got the creature cornered and killed it with an IV pole. I decided then and there to look at snakes outside on the lawn in the future.

We got to know many of the cops pretty well because they were always bringing prisoners and others in to be looked at. Because of the close quarters and the strange people in the ER, we had to have the cops leave their weapons in a lock box like they use in the jail. Before we initiated that, we had a highway patrol officer shot with his own weapon by a drunk in the gurney next to his prisoner's. He was watching his prisoner when the drunk reached out and grabbed his gun, and when he turned around, he was shot fatally in the abdomen.

One cop stood out as one of the toughest men I ever met. He had been on the Chicago Police Force on the night shift and considered our community to be a soft job. One night he was in the ER talking to one of my nurses whose husband was a highway patrol officer when a drunk on one of the gurneys started muttering about how much he hated cops. He got louder and louder and finally leaped at the cop over the intervening gurney. I don't think the cop even broke his conversation but just stuck his fist out and hit the drunk in the jaw knocking him out. After picking up our drunk and getting him squared away, I looked at the cop's gloves. They contained small pockets over the knuckles filled with lead shot.

One of the cops we got to know very well was a woman detective who specialized in juveniles. Everyone knew that if you suspected child abuse, she was the one you called, and she wouldn't give up until she found the truth. One day she came in with a teenage girl in custody and while checking her in, the girl tried to run. The officer grabbed her and suddenly they were on the floor with the detective having her somewhat tight skirt nearly up to her waist and her knee in the teen's back with the teen's arm twisted behind her. There was another officer there and I mentioned how slick she was in controlling this kid. He told me this lady taught hand-to-hand combat in the academy, and since she was very well endowed, the young cadets all thought they could grab her but they always ended up on their backs.

We had a constant problem with child abuse and kept a judge on call 24/7 to obtain custody of a child who we thought was in danger. If we had any suspicion, we had a special mark to put on x-ray orders so that not only was the ordered x-ray taken, but the child would be placed on a large film and a single whole body film would be taken so we could look for old healing fractures as well (a fairly certain sign of child abuse).

One night I had a two-year-old brought in for burns, which the parents said occurred when the child grabbed a cigarette. When I took the child's clothes off, I found a number of obvious cigarette burns on his torso and arms. I went into my office on the pretext of looking up treatment for such a small child and called the police and the judge. The judge gave me custody of the child. I had the nurse clean the wounds and take her time while the cops got there so the parents wouldn't flee with or without the child. When the cops got there, the parents were informed the child was no longer theirs, until a court hearing, and I got the baby admitted and started burn treatment.

Things with the parents got more complicated because they were transients, and it was not clear where the abuse had taken place. Several sheriff's departments, city police, and their specific district attorneys were involved in discussions, each apparently trying to dump the case on someone else. The parents were eventually allowed to leave and I don't know whether they were ever charged. As far as I know, they never tried to get their child back.

Because we were a county facility, we had more than our share of drunks. For the most part they were well behaved and could be controlled because we often had met them time after time. One fellow, however, came in and was uncontrollable. In those days ERs were generally one big room partitioned off with curtains, and this fellow decided he was leaving and walked through every curtain on one side of the room with undressed patients screaming. I followed him out the back door and saw him go across the street and lie down on a bus stop bench. We called the cops. A patrol car pulled up and I pointed to the bench. The officers got out and circled the bench approaching from the back. They stopped and very deliberately pulled on their lead shot weighted gloves before grabbing the sleeping drunk and physically pulling him up off the bench and depositing him in their patrol car.

You could tell very experienced drunks because they would come in requesting chloral hydrate. This was an extremely vile medication, which was the substance used in the original Mickey Finn. It was a liquid that had to be poured over ice for anyone to tolerate it, but it did help with the shakes many of these people had. It was excreted through the lungs, and they claimed the breath of someone on the stuff would attract flies. Judging from the smell, I wouldn't be surprised.

In addition to the drunks, we had the crazies who came in two forms. Some were dangerous but the others were simply crazy, but appeared to be no threat to anyone.

One in particular was a big man who was almost childlike and seemed harmless. One night he was brought in by the cops for a 5150 evaluation. The 5150 referred to a California law that allowed an ER physician or a cop to file a form that placed the subject in a psychiatric facility for three days for evaluation to decide whether he needed long-term psychiatric care. The requirements were that the subject had to be unable to care for himself or he had to be a danger to himself or others.

The man's appearance had changed as he had shaved his head and eyebrows and that, combined with his size (he was around 6'4"), made him appear formidable. The cops said he had been hanging around the late-night bars near the beach and had started following the waitresses home when they went off shift. Not only that, but he also was carrying a large hoe over his shoulder. Naturally the women were concerned and had started calling the cops to take them home when their shifts ended. The cops were tired of being an escort service. I asked the patient why he was carrying a hoe, and he said he was looking for work. He felt he was protecting the waitresses and didn't seem to have any ideas that would result in his harming them. I asked the cops why they brought him in since they could use the 5150 as well as I could, and I couldn't find a good reason to meet the criteria. They admitted they couldn't either and were hoping I could. I advised them they were probably stuck until he found something new to do. I asked the patient to leave the waitresses alone, and he agreed to stop following them but I don't know if he did.

I had had previous experience with this patient when he had cut his thumb and came into the ER holding his thumb in this mouth and blowing into it. I asked him why he was doing that, and he told me since he'd cut himself he was afraid he would deflate. We put an impressive dressing on his thumb after cleaning the minor wound and reassured him that if he left the dressing in place he would heal enough that he would no longer leak.

Traffic accidents were one of the mainstays of the ER. One section of highway just north of us had four lanes but no controlled access. The ocean side of the road had numerous bars and night clubs, so there were people doing left turns, sometimes in a non-too-sober condition across two lanes of oncoming traffic. This resulted in numerous severe accidents. The highway patrol called this area blood alley and tried to patrol it heavily but to only minimal effectiveness.

One Saturday afternoon I had one of the saddest accidents I have witnessed. A man and a woman were brought in by ambulance reportedly the result of a head-on collision. The driver of the other car was left at the scene for the coroner as were the couple's four children. Both of the couple had open fracture dislocations of both knees and had considerable blood loss. As we were getting IVs set up and ordering blood, we called in the orthopedic surgeon on call. He arrived quickly, and we were setting up traction when the man went into cardiac arrest and within minutes the woman also went into arrest. As frequently is the case with trauma arrests, we were unable to resuscitate either of them, and when I thought about the four little bodies in the morgue, I wasn't so sure it was a bad thing. We thought of ourselves as hardened, but a case like that left us depressed for days.

One evening we had a famous Hollywood starlet brought in when she couldn't decide whether to exit the freeway or not and ended up splitting the difference (not a good idea).

She had some minor facial lacerations, which the ER doc would normally have taken care of, but she insisted on having her own Hollywood plastic surgeon drive up and had to wait until her current Hollywood star husband flew in from Vegas. This tied up the ER, and needless to say, the doc on call was very unhappy.

Overdoses were so common we had one gurney set up just for that. In those days we usually caused the patient to vomit, if they were awake, using ipecac. If they were too groggy we'd pass a tube into the stomach and had a large jar of saline on a high shelf, which we'd flush into the stomach, and a "Y" connection, which allowed us to drain the contents of the stomach into a bucket on the floor. The tube we used was very large bore to allow as much of the stomach contents to come up without clogging. We also had to put a tube in the trachea so they couldn't inhale their stomach contents. One such case was a Mexican girl I had met previously when she had an infection. She was brought in unconscious and barely breathing. She had "done a rack of reds." Reds were the street name for homemade Seconol, which was dyed red to try to look like the real thing. These cases were notoriously dangerous because the epiglottis would spasm if disturbed and the patient could suffocate. Because of this, we'd learned to do a "blind" intubation for which you didn't use a laryngoscope but put the tube through the nose and passed it directly into the trachea by feel. You only had one shot because if you missed, they could spasm with fatal results.

I got the tube down and passed the larger tube to wash out any pill fragments left. The patient was then admitted on a respirator. I later went to visit her as she was waking up, and we discussed how close she had come to death. I spent some time with her counseling her about drugs. I didn't see her for a while, and then she turned up in a line of female prisoners the sheriff brought from the jail for routine care. She told me she'd taken advantage of a program they had to stay in jail voluntarily and get clean of drugs. She was then planning on moving to some place like Wyoming where she thought she could avoid her old friends and build a drug-free life. I never saw her again, but I hope it worked for her.

Another drug problem occurred when some wise guy put LSD in the punch at a teen party in a nearby town. There is no treatment for this except to talk them down and try to avoid a "bad trip." We did the best we could with what personnel we had and could borrow from Mental Health. We ended up with about twenty-five confused and frightened teens and about twenty-five sets of angry parents.

At that time we had a lot of problems with insecticides. The workers would come in with nonspecific complaints, and we'd learn they'd been put back into the fields right after they'd been sprayed. They never knew what had been sprayed, and the growers weren't about to admit to this so we generally never knew what the exposure had been. One time, though, we knew specifically what had happened because the problem had come from a DDT manufacturing plant. The worker brought in admitted his respirator didn't fit well because of his beard. These guys were covered with the white powder, which was DDT, and this patient was salivating so severely it was obvious he'd gotten a high dose. The only treatment was a drug called atropine used in very high doses, and that was what we used. When I pushed it IV, the symptoms would correct, but in a short time they would recur so we'd do it again. Eventually he settled down, but I never knew if there were any long-term effects.

As noted previously many of our patients were Mexican field workers and their families. These people were very poor and very polite and grateful for their care. One Saturday night, we'd just about cleaned up the place around midnight when I noticed there was a Mexican family still sitting in the waiting room. I asked my nurse to check and see if they had not known to sign in since we didn't have a chart. She went out and talked with them for a moment and then came back in laughing. It seems they didn't have a TV but had come to the ER waiting room to watch the ambulances and cops come and go instead. They thought it was a pretty good show. I had to admit it would make a great television show and today someone else figured it out as well. We never had the torrid scenes with the nurses however.

Sue and I had been trying unsuccessfully to start a family since my internship, so we had decided to try adoption instead. The agency said there were few white babies available but they could arrange for a black baby fairly readily. We thought about it and decided we had no problems with that because we both felt a baby is a baby so we went ahead with the studies required for adoption in the state of California. The agency called about ten months after our initial inquiry to say they had a baby in northern California and would we like to meet him. I arranged to get some time off and we were set to leave the next day. The next morning was remarkable as we had the alarm set for 6:00 a.m., and it seemed to go off with a vengeance. I woke with the feeling the alarm was shaking the whole house but realized the house really was shaking and we were having an earthquake. Being a Westerner, I had been through a couple of quakes before so I was not very upset. The shaking subsided, but then I was concerned that the hospital might need me. It turned out the quake was centered in San Fernando and all the hospitals in Los Angles were functioning, so we just took back roads to avoid the valley and went ahead to Sacramento. We went to the nursery where they were watching over a baby boy who was to become Douglas. They told us only that his mother was a white college student from the Sacramento area and his father was a black athlete at a major university. That was all the information they were allowed to give out in those days. We were told we could take him then or stay overnight in our motel and pick him up in the morning. Naturally, we weren't going without him so we bought some necessary formula and diapers and went to the motel. That turned out to be a very long night because he was fussy, and the motel had paper thin walls. We didn't want to disturb the other guests so we spent a lot of time walking and holding him.

On the trip home the next day we were going down the freeway when Sue decided Doug needed a new diaper. I asked if she needed me to find a place to pull over, but she said she could just change him in her lap because he was so small. As soon as she had his diaper off, he let go from all orifices, and she was screaming while I was having difficulty holding the car on the road because I was laughing so hard. Having been baptized into motherhood, she had me pull over in the future.

We were a little concerned about how the family would take to a black baby, and when we took some vacation time, we went to my folk's place in Washington State. I wasn't worried about my parents but more about my elderly grandmother who had come from a family whose father was in the KKK. She had told me in the past that the KKK they belonged to didn't worry so much about blacks as they worried about Catholics who they firmly believed had guns stored in the basement of the church and were planning a revolution. When we took Doug to her retirement home, Grandma was so proud of him she took him all over the building to show him off to all her friends. A baby is still a baby regardless of race.

One of the controversies in the residency was abortion. At that time an abortion could be obtained only if the pregnancy was making the mother sick. This included psychiatric illness, and we had a psychiatrist on staff who felt that if a young woman didn't want to be pregnant, then she would naturally have a situational depression and so he would rubber stamp that diagnosis for any young woman planned parenthood or other sources sent to him. The residents were supposed to do these procedures, and I did as expected for a while, but when one of these depressed patients came back to the ER with an overdose after the abortion because she felt so bad about getting it done, I began to rethink my feelings about doing this procedure. Since we'd had to adopt and knew how few infants there were for adoptive parents and since I felt ill after watching small fetal parts flying past in the suction tube on their way to the collecting bag, I decided I didn't want to do any more of these. When I went to the boss with my decision, I discovered there were other residents who felt the same way. He went to the county for advice and was told nobody could be forced to participate in abortions including the OR personnel. We had one junior resident who liked doing the procedure so he took most of them on.

We had a Catholic priest who was the hospital chaplain. Father created quite a few problems for us. He was convinced that since he was a priest, he couldn't transmit or catch disease so he always tried to visit patients in isolation without putting on the gown, gloves, and masks, which were required, which naturally drove the nurses wild. He also figured out the surgical schedule that didn't have abortions explicitly scheduled but were listed as D and C's. He would look on the schedule, and since the women were admitted the night before their surgery, he would make rounds on them telling these good Catholic Mexican girls they were going to go to hell if they proceeded. The resident on at night would end up with crying hysterical young women all over the surgical ward and would have to stop what he was doing to help the nurses to get them settled down.

Our chief resident on my first year had saved up and bought a Porsche sports car, which he was very proud of. One day one of the residents was in a patient room when he heard a crash out in the parking lot. Looking out the window, he saw Father had run into the Porsche. Father looked around, and seeing no one in the parking lot, he drove his car to the other end of the lot and parked. Needless to say the chief resident had a few words for him when he learned what had happened to his pride and joy.

I had a young Mexican field worker come into the ER one day complaining of shortness of breath and tiredness. This kid looked like a male model, and it was hard to believe he had significant shortness of breath, but his blood pressure was unusual in that he was running 100/80, which is a very narrow pulse pressure. I sent him for a chest x-ray thinking it would be normal and we could reassure him. Instead he had a large heart that looked way too round. He had a pericardial effusion. This occurs when fluid is excreted into the sack around the heart called the pericardium. As the pressure on the sack gets higher, the heart is unable to expand and fill normally, so the amount pumped becomes less and less. Unless you relieve this pressure, the patient can die rather quickly. We took the young man to the ICU where I set up to do a pericardiocentesis (put a needle in the pericardium and draw off the fluid). He was on an ECG monitor because if the needle contacted the heart muscle itself, there would appear what is called an injury pattern. The young man really didn't understand what was going on in spite of the efforts of an interpreter, but it was apparent we were serious as we set up a sterile tray and got into gloves and so on. About this time Father came round and saw what we were doing, and since it looked serious to him, he opened his little bag and put on vestments and began giving last rites. The young man didn't understand what we were doing, but he sure understood what Father was doing. His eyes got huge and his heart rhythm became disconnected between the atrium and the ventricle, and I had to have the nurses remove Father until the patient settled down and we could proceed. When the fluid was drained, the patient's color improved and he felt better. We left a catheter in the pericardium to continue drainage. Later the lab told us there were TB organisms in the fluid, and once he was under treatment, the patient improved rapidly.

We had a jail unit on the grounds where prisoners from the county jail who needed inpatient treatment were housed. We also held violent psychiatric patients there. The unit was staffed by one nurse and one deputy sheriff. We had one prisoner who was admitted after he was pulled over by a highway patrol for driving without a license plate on his car. He got out of his car and tried to arrest the highway patrolman for interfering with a federal officer. He assured the cop he was undercover and that was why he had no identification on him and wouldn't tell them his name. At one point he nearly got out of his cell by rushing the deputy bringing him his lunch. Fortunately there was a second deputy there because they were changing shifts. I thought since he used this federal agent routine that maybe he was known to the feds, so I called the local FBI office and asked if they had been having such problems. They said they had but the fellow had been caught and sent to the state mental facility. When I called them, they had to admit their man had escaped the same day this fellow was picked up. They sent a couple of people over to identify him and took him back to the state hospital.

Another incident in the jail unit occurred when a young man who was well known to us as a chronic schizophrenic, who tended to stop his medications, was brought in. In the past there had always been a little scenario we went through to get him to take his medications. He always refused and we always had to threaten to give them as a shot and he always relented and took the pills. Once on his medications he was really a nice fellow. We did not know that since the last time we had seen him, he'd developed some self-confidence, so when we went into his cell and told him he needed to take his pills or we would give them as a shot, he backed into a corner and threw the bedside stand at us and said he wasn't taking a shot either. We were stuck at this point because we couldn't let him get control, so the deputy waded in but the patient caught him in a head lock. The nurse was in the doorway moving back and forth trying to decide whether to give the shot in her hand or to run back to the locked nursing station. I finally got his arm behind his back, and she gave him the shot and he let go of the deputy. After that he was as peaceful as he could be.

Our second year there were only four senior residents since, but our staff was enlarged because we had interns for the first time. This resulted in each of the residents in my class having to be chief resident in one or more specialties. At one time I was chief resident on surgery and on OB at the same time, which meant I left OB to my junior resident and my intern except when a forceps rotation or a C-section was needed. Thus I could avoid routine deliveries of which I had already done plenty.

One day I was called to the ER to evaluate a boy of about twelve for a possible of appendicitis. The story was that he'd been seeing a physician in the barrio who was known for overusing antibiotics (in fact apparently everyone he saw got an injection of some kind). The child had been having pain in the right low abdomen and getting shots for more than a week. This seemed to slow down the progression of his illness but didn't cure anything, so the family finally brought him to the county hospital. His white count was up and he had a little fever, but when I examined him, I didn't find what I thought would be there. He wasn't really tender in his abdomen but seemed to actually hurt over his right hip joint and movement of his hip seemed to be the source of his pain. Hip films didn't help much, but I decided he probably had a septic hip and called the orthopedic consultant on call. He said he was just finishing his office and would be over as soon as he could. Shortly thereafter the child suddenly convulsed and spiked a high fever. He rapidly became short of breath and chest x-ray showed a pattern compatible with staph pneumonia. Staphylococcus is a nasty organism in the lungs and this one was no exception. We started him on antistaph drugs, but the infection rapidly progressed and he died.

The autopsy confirmed he had had a septic hip, which was smoldering along. Finally it broke loose and he had a staph septicemia (blood infection) and seeded his lungs from there. Naturally the family sued the county rather than the fellow in the barrio who had strung this infection along for weeks.

I had one rotation outside the hospital where I spent the mornings in an ENT office and the afternoons in a dermatology office. ENT was fun more because of the special equipment than anything else, but some of their cases were unusual in themselves. We had one cop who had made the mistake of firing his 357 magnum through the window of his car. He immediately became totally deaf, and there wasn't much that could be done but watch over time. He did eventually get most of his hearing back, but he could just as well have never gotten it back.

The afternoons at dermatology were an education in how to make money in medicine. The partner of the man I was following wasn't fifty and was retiring because managing all his apartment buildings was taking too much of his time. They had a number of money-making machines including Grenz ray (low power x-ray) and ultraviolet boxes. They would prescribe so many treatments with these and the patients would come and be put on the machine for a few minutes. They got to bill for this even though they hadn't even seen the patient and a technician was the person who did all the work. The man I followed taught minor plastics at UCLA, and almost everything he did would require tissue transfer, which greatly increased the size of the bill. I even saw him remove a small mole on a lady's behind and create a graft, which was totally unnecessary even for cosmetics. Dermatologists can see a large number of patients in a day because most of the time you know what the problem is immediately, and if you don't, you'll probably have to biopsy the lesion. If you haven't seen the condition before, you will never get the diagnosis, so it was a good rotation for me to get to see a lot of pathology in a very short period of time.

Another rotation that was somewhat different was in Public Health. We would go with the county sanitarian to inspect restaurants and check swimming pools at motels. Sometimes even the nicest-looking restaurant would have numerous violations when you got behind the counter. When we went into the restaurant, he would run around like crazy putting thermometers in steam tables, cooling cabinets, and refrigerators because the owners would try to change the temperatures if they could. It's always cheaper to keep your steam table cooler than is safe and your cooler warmer than is safe. After inspecting a number of restaurants, I quit eating out for a month. One place even had a structural problem, which would have been very expensive to change so they just took a hit each inspection. They had a heated pass-through from the kitchen below, which was a cooled glass case for pies. The case was warmed by the infrared lights over the pass-through and was always too warm for the cream pies there. This increased the chance of bacterial growth.

We went with the Public Health nurses on their rounds around the county. At one place the nurse warned me to watch the back of the trailer home as we pulled in. Two men ran out the back when our county car became visible. We went in to check on two women with new babies and see how they were doing with nutrition and baby care. The nurse later explained that the men running out the back lived there, but when they saw a county car, they would run away because the women were getting support on a program for mothers and babies and there were not supposed to be men living there. They couldn't tell if we were with the Welfare Department, so they ran and hid when we drove up.

We also helped out in the Public Health clinics. Some were traveling birth control clinics that were held in places like church basements and the like. The ones in the affluent parts of the county were well attended by well-dressed young women that one would not normally expect to be at a welfare clinic. One woman I was examining had a large bruise on her buttock, and I asked her what had happened. She told me she fell cleaning her pool. The nurse told me that these people were trying to look like they were doing well and had pools and country club memberships but were stretched so thin they came to the welfare clinics because they didn't have money for birth control. I always felt this was cheating, especially when I couldn't afford a pool.

One of the services we would perform was placing IUDs (intra-uterine devices for birth control). The nurses were so enamored of IUDs that they tied the tails of a standard IUD through their pierced ears and wore them as earrings. One time I had just finished putting one in, when the lady had a massive vagal response to the placement. When this happens, their heart rate slows severely, and their blood pressure drops, and they can convulse, which she did. I asked the nurse for the medication I needed to block this reaction only to discover they brought nothing with them. I had to get one nurse on each side and have them hold her while I got a speculum into the vagina and managed to get hold of the string and remove the IUD, which allowed the patient to recover. After that I arranged for a special package of drugs for resuscitation to go to those clinics before another incident occurred. I was quite angry that the people who planned these clinics had never thought of this.

There was also a clinic in the barrio in the next town where people could be seen for various problems. The nurses worked particularly on pregnancy and infant nutrition, but when the resident was there, they could see anything that came in. The nurses had to go out on the street and see to it that everybody knew which car belonged to the resident, so we didn't come out to find our cars stripped. A friend of mine who did a residency in Chicago told me they had the same thing, but the nurses didn't hit the street fast enough and they found his car up on blocks. They told him not to worry about it, and sure enough when he went out at the end of the day, his car had wheels back on and with brand-new tires. He told me he was afraid to ask where they came from. Generally poor people are very grateful for such clinics and the free care they provide and try to look out for the people working there so they will continue to return.

One night I was in the ER when the ambulance brought in a three- or four-year-old child who had been hit by a truck. His height was such that the truck's bumper was even with his head, which had taken all the force. He had sustained obvious severe brain injuries and we sent for the neurosurgeon on call who arrived very quickly. He barely looked at the child and wanted to go right to the OR. I had anticipated this and called in the crew, but the anesthesiologist on call was out to dinner with his wife in the far end of the county and would take at least thirty minutes to arrive. The neurosurgeon said we didn't have that much time since the problem was rapidly getting worse, and the only chance the child had was if he had an epidural bleed. He looked at me and said, "You are a senior resident, aren't you, and you've had anesthesia rotations, so get up to the OR and put this child to sleep." I had the ER nurse call in my backup and with great trepidation went to the OR. I had to intubate the child, and he had a broken jaw so that when I got him into position, all I could see in his throat was blood. I aimed at the place where I could see the bubbles coming from in the blood in his throat and managed to get him intubated. The neurosurgeon was proceeding rapidly while I went ahead with the induction, which I wasn't even sure was necessary since child was so far gone. When he had drilled the holes in the skull, all he found was bloody mush instead of brain. By that time the anesthesiologist arrived and I could go back to the ER. They could do nothing so they closed and allowed the child to die.

Another problem came up when I was senior resident on Peds. We had several hired docs working in the outpatient clinics, and one of them asked if I would come down and evaluate a child with headaches. The child was about ten years old, and the story obtained through an interpreter was that he'd been having increasingly strong headaches for the past couple months. The mother had taken him several places, but no one could diagnose the source of these headaches. The only other history of interest was that as an infant he had TB meningitis treated in San Diego with good results. When I examined the child, I found he had severe papilledema in his eye grounds. This is a swelling in the retina when it is being pushed forward by increased intracranial pressure pushing the retinal nerve forward. I admitted the child and called the neurosurgeon on call to see him. He agreed that there was a severe intracranial pressure increase and thought it was secondary to scar from the meningitis blocking the normal circulation and drainage of the cerebral-spinal fluid. Because it was late Friday afternoon, he felt it could wait the weekend and scheduled the child for surgery Monday morning. When we made rounds Saturday morning the child looked about the same but suddenly went into convulsions and died. The neurosurgeon was there with us, but we couldn't do anything fast enough to do any good. The pressure had finally pushed the brain stem into the spinal canal. I think both the neurosurgeon and I learned a lesson from this, but it was a lousy teaching experience.

We had hired docs working in the outpatient clinics, and one of them did this because he wasn't up to private practice because he had severe asthma. We had learned the asthma seemed to be triggered by drinking and he was an alcoholic. When he didn't show up for work at the clinic in the morning, we would send the ambulance out to his apartment and they would break the door down. They told me they would generally find him on the floor barely breathing surrounded by epinephrine (adrenaline) syringes and foil wraps from aminophylline suppositories. When he came in, we always had to intubate him, and since he'd already used maxi doses of our usual drugs, we would have to find a vein and push steroids IV to break the attack. He told me once he'd lost his apartment and had to move because the landlord got tired of fixing the door. One Monday he failed to show up for work, and the ambulance was sent out, but he had apparently had his drinking episode Friday night and they were way too late.

Our hospital was on a campus of county buildings, which included the welfare office. One day I was in the ER when a man came running in saying there was a man at the welfare office with his abdomen wide open and his intestines falling out. We took a gurney out of the ER and rolled it over to the welfare office to find the scene exactly as described except for the hysterical wife. The story was that the man had had surgery for cancer and just had his stitches removed in surgery clinic. He'd gone to get his welfare check when the entire wound opened up. We covered him with sterile sheets and sent him up to surgery where after a thorough cleaning he was reclosed. He probably hadn't healed properly because of his cancer.

We had a new anesthetic called Ketamine become available while I was in residency. This has since been relegated to the veterinary market but it originally was available for humans. I had a young man come in with a leg fracture and decided to try it in the ER. Since it was an injection and fairly short lived, it was felt safe to use for short anesthetics such as setting fractures. The only negative with this drug was its tendency to lower seizure thresholds. We gave him the anesthetic and after some struggle got the fracture reduced. I was starting to apply the cast when the large ventilating fan outside the room kicked in. The noise was apparently too much, and the patient immediately went into convulsions, which totally disrupted the reduction I had worked so hard to set. The seizures didn't last long, and we went back to our old technique of admitting him to surgery and setting his fracture there under general anesthesia.

Our Ortho clinic also had a new casting substance, which was fiberglass. This wasn't the fiberglass used today, which sets with the use of water very much like plaster, but was UV sensitive, so that when you had the cast done the way you wanted, you put it into a light box and it hardened almost immediately. This was wonderful as it put you under no time pressure when applying a complicated cast, but it had the interesting side effect of changing the rules in the local high school football league. Since the cast wouldn't break, a kid with a forearm cast could still play. Unfortunately the kids learned early that the cast made a great club, and the league had to make a rule that if playing with a cast, it must have two inches of foam rubber over it.

One day we had a lady come into the ER complaining of several hours of severe abdominal pain. She was morbidly obese, weighing well over three hundred pounds. Her abdominal exam was no help because I couldn't feel anything through all the fat. She gave a history of not having had a period for over a year, which is not unusual for obese women because estrogen is fat soluble and so much is stored they can't get the sharp changes in estrogen-progesterone ratios necessary to have periods. When I went to do a pelvic exam, my finger ran into a smooth, hard mass, which turned out to be a baby's head. The patient was in labor and getting close to delivery and hadn't the vaguest idea she was even pregnant. This was the source of her abdominal pain. This case eventually turned into a nightmare because the baby got stuck. The junior resident in OB called me at home, but since I'd worked in the ER all day the day before and had been up all night and worked another full day, I had been working for thirty-six hours straight. I told him to call the attending as I didn't feel I was safe any longer. He did, and they had a terrible time getting the baby delivered. Apparently the babe had been stuck with ruptured membranes for some time, and the infant was septic and subsequently died in the nursery. There was a lawsuit and after I had started in private practice two lawyers flew up from LA and tried to get me to say things were done poorly. They had named me in the suit since my name was in the chart, and they intimated they would remove me from the suit if I would help them out. I refused and refused to speculate on why things were done the way they were since I hadn't been there. I was eventually removed from the suit anyway.

One of the rotations of my senior year was to precept with a gastroenterologist who was generally conceded to be the best internist in town. This man had started with the residency with a great deal of doubt whether Family Practice residents could do all the things we were expected to do but had been slowly won over. In fact he eventually became the residency director when he left private practice. It was very sad that he was forced out of private practice because his reputation was so good that he was always consulted on the most difficult cases, and these were the ones, which had a higher percentage of bad outcomes and he was named in all the suits, which resulted from bad outcomes without regard to whether there was bad medicine. He finally got tired of all the time in court and left private practice. The lawyers had forced the best man in town out of business.

One of my responsibilities was to write orders on patients the gastroenterologist was asked to consult on. There was one surgeon who apparently couldn't or wouldn't write his own fluid orders, so I went every day and wrote the next day's fluid orders on his post ops. My preceptor would read the orders later and countersign them since this was in the private hospital in town. The surgeon didn't understand electrolytes and got upset with me for not getting a new set of labs every day. I was simply watching intake and output and writing orders accordingly, but when he challenged me, I bet him the electrolytes were perfect and we drew a set. They were perfect and he never bothered me again.

We got called to look at a woman in the ICU who had had surgery scheduled but after a dose of pre-op Demerol had quit breathing and had never restarted. There was a mass on her chest x-ray, which was why they had scheduled the surgery, and it became apparent after examining her, that this was probably a tumor called a thymoma, which is associated with myasthenia gravis. We suggested they go ahead and remove the tumor which they did, but the poor woman didn't start breathing on her own for several weeks in spite of medications.

The other new experience for me was to mix a patient's chemotherapy. Chemo was in its infancy, and we used very toxic substances. This patient was getting mustard, which was the substance from which mustard gas was produced during World War 1. You had to mix it from vials under a negative pressure hood, and you had to wear heavy gloves, face shield, and a special apron. If you spilled even a drop, you were in trouble. I got through it but it sure made me nervous. I couldn't imagine having that stuff pushed into my vein.

One of the more important lessons I had to learn was that the buck often stops with the patient's primary care physician. I had a gentleman who came in having chest pain and had an acute heart attack shown on his ECG. After he'd been in the ICU a day or so, he started to complain of severe pain in his leg. When I looked, I found his leg was pale and cold and had no pulses. I called the vascular surgeon to look. He agreed the patient had clotted off his femoral artery and needed immediate surgery to save his leg and eventually his life. The cardiologist I had consulted on the case informed me that if the patient had to undergo surgery, he would die from the anesthetic, and cited an article claiming 100 percent fatality in the immediate post-heart attack period. I finally forced a compromise by getting the surgeon to open the artery and fish out the clots under local anesthetic in the ICU, which went wonderfully. Unfortunately the patient had a massive stroke a few days later, and died anyway, but the lesson of having to decide and guide a patient caught between specialists continued to be a problem throughout my career. Looking back, I suspect this patient had a hyper coagulation disorder, but we weren't very aware of these in those days.

Next to the hospital on the county campus was the county psych unit, which had a small population of inpatients. We were responsible for medical care of these people and would get called over if a problem developed. A fairly common call was a code blue when they had over medicated a patient for electroshock therapy. When we arrived, we would find a patient who wasn't breathing but had a good heart beat and blood pressure. Most of these patients needed simply to be reminded to breath. Often I would stand there and tell the patient to take a breath, which he would do, but he had to be told each time until the medication wore off or was reversed.

One day I was called to psych to evaluate a patient who had been admitted the night before and was no longer responsive. When I arrived, I found a patient lying in bed and not moving. He had very course hair and a swelling known as myxedema. This was typical of a patient with severe hypothyroidism. He still had the Thorazine capsule on his tongue he had been given the night before. It was apparent they had admitted a case of myxedema madness, which is well described in the literature. We transferred the patient to the ICU and started IV Tri-iodothyronine, which is the fastest-acting form of thyroid. Lab results confirmed our initial diagnosis but we were too late and the patient went ahead and died shortly after admission.

There was a huge man employed by the psych unit as an aid whose responsibility was controlling violent patients. This man stood about 6'4" and weighed about 300 pounds. One night he came into the ER with an ambulance with two injured men. It turned out these two idiots tried to mug him while he was walking on the beach. He'd simply thrown them both headfirst into a sand dune.

Having responsibility for the jail was sometimes a problem. The hospital had better food and was also easier to escape from, so the inmates would try all sorts of ploys to get admitted. One fellow showed up with the smell of chlorine on his breath claiming to have tried to commit suicide by eating the cleanser they had been using on a cleanup detail. We couldn't be sure how much material he had ingested, if any, so we had to treat him. The recommended treatment was to drink a substance with fat in it to avoid absorption. We sent to the kitchen and got a quart of half and half, which we made him drink down. He was then watched for a period of time and sent back to the jail. These men were kept in a tank with up to twenty other inmates and a single toilet, which was flushed by the guards from outside the tank. We explained to the guards not to be in a hurry since we were pretty sure this fellow would develop stiatorrhea, which occurs when you have too much fat to absorb and results in severely stinky stools. We suspected the other inmates would cure him of any further fake overdoses. I don't know if it worked, but we didn't have any more ingestions.

Our chief resident sent one inmate back to the jail with a gut full of broken razor blades after talking to a buddy of his who was at LA County. His friend said they'd had an epidemic of this and after observing a large number of them had found this didn't cause a problem surprisingly passing on through. The x-ray sure was impressive, however.

We had one older black inmate who was brought over because of a swollen knee. We were already familiar with him because we'd seen his knee before and it was thought he had a brown synovitis caused by repeated trauma to his knee. He was a fry cook and would close the drawers below his work surface with that knee. The orthopedic surgeon had wanted to operate on his knee before, but he couldn't take the time off work. Since he was going to be off work regardless because he was in jail, he thought it would be a good time to get his knee fixed. I asked him what he'd been convicted of, and he said receiving stolen property. He claimed he had no idea those twenty typewriters some guy sold him cheap were stolen, and of course, I certainly believed him.

At surgery we found the excess synovium we had expected, and it was excised. As we were closing the orthopedic surgeon decided to put some steroids into the joint to suppress further inflammation. The next day his knee was swollen, and he had a little fever. Shortly after, the pathologist called to say he'd found coccidiomycosis in the synovium. This organism causes San Joaquin Valley Fever, which usually is a flu-like illness contracted when you inhale the dust in the valley. In black people, however, it was a different story because blacks and American Indians seem not to have good immunity and can have complications such as this man had. The steroid had decreased his ability to fight the infection, which was why he had the fever and inflammation. I started him on the only treatment we had and fortunately he responded very well.

Coccidiomycosis has to go through a phase in the dust to develop infective spores, so it generally is not transmitted from person to person, but I had a patient with the one form that can undergo person-to-person spread. This patient was a thirty-year-old black man who had a skin infection. Because it's on the outside, it can go through its spore developing form right there on the surface of the skin. I think he got me because after caring for him, I developed some lymph nodes in my chest but I wasn't sick and my TB test remained negative. He had been sent to Chino (where there is a California state prison) for heroin use and sale and contracted the disease there. He'd had two courses of Amphotericin B before ending up in our facility. I always thought this was cruel and unusual punishment to send black prisoners to a coccidiomycosis area. I felt badly for him because the one thing in the entire world he wanted was to ride horses, which I'm pretty sure was never going to happen. It was always a race with amphotericin whether you were going to kill the fungus or the patient's kidneys first, and this was even worse with multiple courses but we managed to get him through it.

Addicts were always a problem in the ER, but some were more memorable than others. One Saturday I had a mother bring in her twelve-year-old daughter requesting pain medication for the daughter's rotten teeth. When I looked at the daughter she did indeed have rotten teeth with deep cavities and was obviously in pain. I offered several remedies, but the mother was quite insistent that the only thing that helped was a drug called Talwin. This drug had come on the market claiming to be non-addicting but had proved on the contrary to be very addicting, and I immediately became suspicious of the situation. I gave the girl a local anesthetic and a very small number of Talwin, but on Monday, I checked with the local dentists and found the mother would show up in their offices on a walk-in basis at the end of the day and convince them to give enough Talwin until they could set up an appointment. Further investigation found this woman had originated in Seattle and worked her way south. I was called later that day by a pharmacist asking how many Talwin I had given the girl and when I told him ten, he said he had a prescription for a hundred. We notified the police who caught the mother at the pharmacy and arrested her. I hope someone finally took care of the girl's teeth because I really think they were hurting but never being treated, so the mother could hang on to her drug ticket.

Addicts never knew exactly what they were injecting, and sometimes some heroin would appear on the street in a form that hadn't been cut as much as they were used to and they would get what they called a hot shot, which could prove fatal. For some reason they had developed some strange remedies for this, possibly based on the use of fats to slow absorption from the stomach in some overdoses. They would try to inject either mayonnaise or milk to counteract the shot. Fortunately they seldom were able to get these into the vein, but they would get a nasty sterile abscess at the site of the attempted injection. If they hit the vein, they would get multiple fat emboli to their lungs, which could kill them as well.

Most of the prisoners in the jail unit were addicts who fed their habit by illegal means. I quickly learned that much of the crime on the streets was drug related either selling drugs or stealing or prostituting to get money for drugs. One prisoner seemed way too comfortable after being in the jail unit several days. I told the deputy he seemed to have a source inside the unit, and we agreed on a shakedown of his cell. We found nothing, but as things were being put back I noticed a ratty pack of cigarettes. When we looked in the pack, we found there were cigarettes in the front but capsules hidden in the back. The deputy didn't want to do the paperwork to file charges so he just took them away. The prisoner claimed they were just pain pills, but I knew this was unlikely so I tried the thing I'd seen on TV of putting a tiny amount of the powder on my tongue. We flushed the capsules, but as I was leaving, I suddenly I knew what the powder was. My tongue had gone numb and I realized the powder was cocaine, which we used as a local anesthetic for nasal procedures. I decided not to use the taste test again.

One young couple came in requesting admission to help them kick a heroin habit. They told me they both had reached the point where their habits required over $200 a day. They couldn't steal enough, and she couldn't turn enough tricks to pay this much. After they were there a couple days, they both appeared more comfortable than I would have expected. I walked into his room one morning to find them kissing but things did not look normal. When I forced him to open his mouth, I found she had been passing him a pill. After some discussion I realized they had come in to decrease their habit so they could afford it, not to kick the habit altogether. I discharged them both.

As the second year of residency came to a close, I received my active duty orders from the air force. They had sent me a form asking where in the country I would prefer to be stationed, and I had told them that since we had a transracial adoption, I would prefer not to be stationed in the Deep South where some states still made families like mine illegal. They assigned me in a western state instead and we started packing.

Air Force

When I got my active duty orders, we went out to my new base and met the hospital commander. We also went looking for a house because we had decided that getting a tax-free housing allowance and being able to deduct the interest payments would be way ahead of living in base housing. We then went back to the residency and packed our U-Haul. While Susan was getting settled in, I had to go to medical basic training for physicians, nurses, and dentists.

Medical basic was held at Shepherd Air Force Base near the Texas-Oklahoma line. This is not really a scenic area, and the instructors weren't enamored of the place. One instructor warned us that if we ate off base, there would be a lot of flies but not to swat them because they were the state bird of Texas. The jokes went on and on.

I was housed with two dentists who had never had any experience with the military. I had been in Army ROTC in college so had some minimal experience. I had purchased my uniforms from another doc who was getting out so didn't have to spend a lot of time and money taking care of that. We were told we would be required to attend a formal dining in, so we had to go to one of the two tailors just off base to get the required formal uniforms (short white coat with tux pants and tux shirt). These guys had a racket because there was no one else, and we wouldn't wear this again. I did wear it once in the next two years, about which there will be more later.

We were also told we would have to march in review for inspection and had to have a spit shine on our shoes. My two dentist roommates worked all evening trying to get a spit polish shine on their shoes, and I spent about fifteen minutes. They were amazed when they saw my shoes, so I took pity on them and told them I had learned while in ROTC from a former marine drill sergeant how to put a thick coating of wax on the toe of the shoe and then melt it with your Zippo lighter. A little buffing and you were done.

One evening we were walking back to our barracks after dinner when I noticed a number of the new medical officers crossing the street in front of me. They would then cross back further down. There was one man walking toward me, and when I got closer, I could see he was a chief master sergeant and really looked the part with a face of leather and deep wrinkles and hash marks (stripes on the lower sleeve marking number of years on duty) almost up to his elbows. The officers were so unsure of saluting protocol they were crossing the street to avoid saluting him. I just waited for him to salute first and returned his salute and kept on walking while he was smiling at the young officers afraid of him.

After a couple weeks of lectures, I got pulled out of class by a full colonel and told there were only three of us who had Family Practice residency training and I was the only one who had completed the entire program. He had decided I would be ideal to stay at Shepard and teach the physician's assistance program. I went into a panic because my base was a much nicer place to live, so I called my hospital commander to ask what I could do. He asked if we had bought the house we were looking at, and when I said we had, he recommended that I tell the people at Shepard we had done so and would incur a financial hardship to move at this late date. They were very understanding and called one of the other family practitioners out of class.

The docs got lucky one time. We had been scheduled for bivouac one day, but the dentists and nurses were sent without the docs because the military was having problems with drug use in Vietnam and they wanted to go over new medical regs on how to handle drug users. After a morning of lectures we were bused out to the bivouac site to find the dentists and nurses looking like they had been dragged through a knothole. They had spent the 105-degree morning running the obstacle course carrying stretchers.

We did have to learn the one man fireman's carry, but other than that, we spent the afternoon in demonstrations of the different kinds of wounds different firearms would cause. We then got to spend the evening in an emergency drill with a mock airplane crash. They had an old aircraft hull there and drums in which they burned oil-soaked rags. As things went along, the instructors were throwing flash-bangs to keep things interesting. Some of the people had family along, and they got to sit in a set of stands and watch. I was given a death mask and told to lie down in the grass and play dead, which suited my acting abilities to a tee.

We passed in review the next morning and had the formal dining—in (an old British custom with very formal rules) that night, and we were considered fully trained medical officers. On the flight back I had to change planes at Tulsa, and while sitting in the waiting room to start boarding my next flight, I noticed a large man in a gray suit approach the desk clerk. When I looked around, we were surrounded by similar men. They announced there had been a bomb threat on our plane, and the men were FBI and Sky Marshals. We were moved to the end of the building and the plane was brought round and the luggage was taken off. We were told to find our own bags and stand by them. They then moved the plane to the far side of the airport to search it, and one group of the agents started looking through our bags. When they got to mine, the first one they opened had my uniforms in it with captain's bars on the shoulders. The agent asked if I was an active duty military officer, and when I said I was, he said we won't need to search your bags. I told him that was fine, but I knew there were kooks in the military too and please search all bags. I realized later that I probably outranked him, and they didn't want trouble. We then waited until we should have reached our destination, and when nothing happened, they brought the plane back and reloaded the bags and us. I wished they had given us another plane in case they'd missed something.

The hospital and clinic at our base was a collection of WWII temporary barracks stuck end to end or end to side. Each separate building was level, but if they didn't match, a ramp was placed going up or down as needed. We had about twenty inpatient beds and another four ICU beds. My job was to be chief of General Therapy and director of Emergency Services. This slot was for a lieutenant colonel, and I was a captain but was promoted to (brevet) major in a few months. I had four general medical officers (MDs right out of internship) and one internal medicine specialist. I was supposed to have eight GMOs. I was to see patients the same as the GMOs and also manage the schedules for the MOD (Medical Officer of the Day) who ran the ER at night and make decisions on sending physicians with the crash wagon if necessary. We had two crash wagons (large four wheel-driven ambulances) and two cosmopolitans (ambulances like a hearse), which we dispatched as needed. I also managed day-to-day issues in the clinic with the help of my clinic nurse (a lieutenant colonel) and my top sergeant.

Our schedule was to see walk-in active duty personnel (sick call) from 0700 to 0900, and the rest of the day was spent seeing appointments, mostly with dependents and retirees. There was a large retiree population living near the base, and they got their medical care free for life.

Shortly after I had arrived, one of my corpsmen complained that when he'd walked past the defibrillator in the ER, it jumped a spark about a foot between the paddles, which were stored on top. I went to investigate and discovered the defibrillator was an ancient AC unit, which hadn't been used in medicine for years. I immediately went to my boss, the hospital commander, and advised him we had to replace it as well as the one in the ICU because they were dangerous both to patients and personnel. This was done, but I got ribbed by the chief of dentistry about taking his new dental chair because the money used to replace the defibrillators was taken from money in his budget for a new dental chair.

One of our regular patients, an elderly lady who was the widow of a WWI corporal killed in action, was trying to live on his pension. She received a lot of help from the Mormon Church even though she wasn't a member, but her husband had been. She was notorious for bringing baked goods for the doctors, but the physicians who had left warned me her hygiene wasn't so good. Her first visit she brought me an angel food cake but when I looked it over, I found a used corn plaster stuck to the underside, so I removed it and sent the cake to the corpsmen's barracks.

We had a number of corpsmen and their skills varied widely. The senior sergeants were very knowledgeable, and some of them had been in the situation where they were the only medical care, such as a snowed in DEW line radar station. Since most of their training was expected to be on the job, the young men just out of the corpsmen's school were not very useful, and I explained to new ones as they arrived that if they heard a "code blue" called on the loud speakers, they were to back up to a wall and stand there unless a doctor or NCO told them otherwise.

When I arrived, I inherited a legal case from the outgoing internist. This was a lady who was waiting Medevac to another base where her husband had been assigned. She had had a stroke, and one side of her body didn't work very well but she could get around. The story was that she had been having headaches, and after several visits to the internist, she had a major stroke. She had been on birth control pills, and no one had asked so she'd continued to take them. She told me she and her husband were having problems, and she had gone to see a lawyer about divorce and had left his office with a malpractice suit against the Air Force instead.

Not long after I'd started at the base, I was on MOD when a young man was brought in by his mother after an injury in youth football. The exam was pretty benign, but I ordered an x-ray for thoroughness and to reassure the mother. The x-ray techs were on call in the evening from their nearby barracks and were supposed to come in only when called. This evening the call was a tech sergeant who had an attitude. He came in and took the x-ray, but then when he brought the patient back to the waiting room, he proceeded to tell me an x-ray was not needed, and air force doctors didn't know what they were doing. He did all this in a waiting room full of patients. I suppose he thought he could intimidate me so I wouldn't call him at night. His mistake was that I wasn't a GMO but had completed residency in a county hospital and wasn't easily intimidated. I called him into a back room and told him his attitude was totally unacceptable. I ordered him to meet me at the hospital commander's office at 0700 where we'd discuss it. In the morning I explained to the colonel what had happened and then had to convince him to leave the sergeant with his stripes. Instead he was offered an Article 15 (discipline without court martial), and of course he accepted. He was put on probation for his stripe, fined $300 and confined to barracks for six weeks. The rest of the time I was there he was polite but certainly not friendly. He eventually got busted when he was assigned to Vietnam, went on a binge, and missed his port call.

I had one sergeant who was our official scrounger, and if we needed something in the clinic, he would find a way to get it. One day he came into my office with a pile of prescriptions with things like Tylenol and Sudafed on them. He told me he used these to barter with the civilian workmen since they could get these free from our pharmacy if they had an official Air Force prescription. One day he told me to take a look at our command room. The command room was off the ER and housed a couple radios connected to the base tower and fire department as well as dedicated telephones one of which (the red one) we knew nothing about except it would ring once a day for a line check. I always assumed it connected to NORAD. When I went into the command room, I discovered it had new walnut paneling. The sergeant told me to keep the generals out of there because they might get suspicious when they found the paneling was the same as the new paneling in the Officers' Club Command Bar. Since someone had misfigured, and they'd been a little short of paneling at the Officers' Club and had had to order more. We also got some very nice planters built in the waiting room one day.

One of my duties was to decide if an incident requiring the presence of a crash wagon was severe enough to send a flight surgeon, or if the corpsmen could handle it. Most of the time they would go and sit alongside the runway until the incident was over and then return. We had a daily courier plane, an old Goony bird from WWII, which frequently had one engine out but could fly just fine on three, and we were constantly scrambling the crash wagon with only the corpsmen aboard. One day we got the call from the tower that they were coming in with their control compromised. The story we learned later was that there were seventeen passengers, which was not uncommon, because if the plane had room, you could "catch a hop" from one base to another for free. There were no seats on these craft so people just sat on the floor and leaned against the bulkhead. This time someone had tried to get up to walk around and reached up to grab something to pull himself up and grabbed the release on a twenty-man life raft, which inflated. This left the people all pressed against the sides of the aircraft, so some genius got the cargo door open and they pushed the life raft out. Now these planes had control cables running along the fuselage, and of course the raft caught on one so the pilot was trying to fly the airplane with a twenty-man life raft flapping on the controls, making it very hard to control the aircraft. We scrambled a physician with the crash wagon that time although they landed without incident. The ambulance crew told me they were afraid they'd have to bring in the guy who pulled the cord if the pilot ever caught him.

The tower guys didn't know how little we knew about airplanes, so sometimes communications left something to be desired. One day we were called by the tower that they had a marine trainer plane coming in with two engines out. My sergeant and I looked at each other and got on the radio to ask how many engines this plane had. The tower replied two, which meant the plane was coming in without power. We scrambled a flight surgeon on that one too.

We had a recon plane, which at that time was very hush-hush, land one day without power, and we had to check out the pilot. He told us he'd had a flameout over Whitehorse, and we were the first base he could get down to. Even so he'd circled over the nearby area to lose speed and knocked out a number of windows in the town with his sonic boom. A couple of the docs went over to look at this aircraft and got to see it before command remembered this was top secret and put a guard on it.

Since this was during the Vietnam conflict, we were seeing people coming back with what today would be called PTSD, but that was a diagnosis we didn't have at that time. I remember one marine captain who came in with headaches so severe he'd been pulled from the line and sent back to the states for workup. Even though all tests were normal, he was convinced he had a brain cancer and was in my office pleading to be released back to combat because he said he'd rather die with a bullet in his head than of a brain cancer. We had to transfer him to a navy hospital with psychiatric services.

Another time I had a staff sergeant come in who had been sent back from his fourth tour in Vietnam because he'd become "kill crazy," meaning he'd quit differentiating between friend and foe and was willing to kill everybody. He came into my office smelling strongly of alcohol and talking about how he wanted to kill someone in uniform. I kind of buttoned up my white coat so the uniform didn't show so much. When I got up to go to the door to get some help, he trapped me against the wall with his hands on my throat, telling me how easy it would be for him to kill me. I finally got back behind my desk and talked him into seeing the base psychiatrist. I called the psychiatrist and told him I had a man who was very upset and needed him to come down. The psych said he was very busy and to get him an appointment. I said, "You don't understand. This man's *VERYUPSET*," but he still didn't get it, so I told the patient he needed some medication to help with his nerves, and when I got him to agree, I called the corpsman at the front and ordered him to bring a syringe with a hundred milligrams of Thorazine down for this patient. I think the size of the dose got his attention, and he told me later he'd brought two other corpsmen with him who waited just outside in the hall. I was a little afraid the dose might damage the patient, but at that point I really didn't care. The medication knocked him out, and we moved him to a locked cell on the inpatient side. I learned later the civilian police were looking for him because just before coming in, he'd broken both his father-in-law's legs. I later called the psychiatrist and told him I thought he was the most unperceptive psychiatrist I'd ever met. He apoligized.

Our base was located at the foot of the mountains and skiing was very popular. We had so many ski injuries the orthopedic surgeon (we only had one) bought a binding tester and held binding clinic every Friday afternoon. In spite of this the fractures and sprains would pile up in the ER, so he set a time on Saturday and Sunday when he would come in and take care of the ones the MOD couldn't handle. One day we had a call from one of the nearby resorts that they had an active duty airman who had fallen and had his ski break and go through his leg. I set off with two corpsmen in the cosmopolitan to pick him up. When we arrived, the ski shop had done as I'd requested and cut the remainder of the ski down so he could be handled. I didn't want to remove the rest of the ski in the field in case he started to bleed heavily. We got a dressing on the wound and started down the mountain. I was in the passenger seat when the corpsman driving asked quietly whether I had hold of the handle to the door. I asked why and he said because the brakes were out and I needed to be ready to jump. We made it down the mountain on the gears but it was exciting.

Because we were so close to the skiing resorts, we were chosen to host the All Air Force Skiing competition. This included the usual downhill and slalom courses and resulted in some of the worst fractures we had seen. The competitors would tighten their bindings as tight as possible so their skis wouldn't come off from the forces they would generate, but it also meant they wouldn't release when they were supposed to when they fell. That long ski bouncing around really did a job on their legs.

We even had injuries from the slopes from non-skiers. One day I was in the ER when they brought in a little six-year-old girl. The girl was the daughter of an enlisted man who had been killed in Vietnam. The mother told me they couldn't afford to ski but went up sometimes to watch. The girl had been near the Bunny Slope when one of the kids coming down was not able to stop. The kid had put his pole out front and it stuck in the little girl's chest. Unfortunately they had removed the ski pole on the slope before coming in so we were going to have trouble seeing where it had gone. The exam showed a hole just to the left of the sternum right over the heart. The chest x-ray showed a tented structure pulled away from the heart, which I realized was the pericardium (the lining around the heart. The ECG didn't show an injury pattern, so I called the civilian chest surgeon in the nearby city and we agreed to transfer her there for observation both for bleeding and infection of the mediastinum (middle of the chest). She did well on antibiotics and went home soon. I guess it depended how you looked at it: she was either very lucky or very unlucky.

I had another six-year-old brought in one time whose family had sent him out to water their stallion. The stallion had bit him on the face, and when I removed the dressings, I found the skin from his throat to just below his eye was gone. It was obvious we weren't equipped to treat this wound, and I explained to the parents it would require skin grafting. I talked to one of the plastic surgeons in town and learned it was worse than I had thought because it was in the area he would one day grow a beard so they would have to swing flaps from areas with beard-producing tissue and then flaps from the flaps until it was all covered. He felt the child was probably in for years of surgery. I'm afraid I had little sympathy for the family who had sent a six-year-old out to care for a dangerous animal.

Another family brought in an eighteen-month baby who had had a pacifier tied to her neck with a ribbon. She apparently had gotten her pacifier caught on the side of the crib and then lost her balance thereby hanging herself. The parents had found her hanging and rushed her into the hospital. We found tiny red spots on her face and eyes, which are called petechiae and are the result of tiny blood vessels breaking when hanging. The parents must have gotten there barely in time. We admitted the child for observation and sent protective services to check the home and make sure this wasn't the result of abuse.

We had another incident with one of the cosmopolitans. This time it was the one that doubled as the hospital commander's staff car. We had two corpsmen who were national guards and did their weekend active duty with us. We'd sent them into town to pick up blood from the blood bank. These fellows were professional ambulance drivers in civilian life, which probably saved their lives. They called on the radio to tell us they were on their way back in heavy traffic when the left front wheel just came off. They were able to hold the ambulance in their lane and get stopped and we sent the tow truck from the motor pool to bring them in. The hospital commander just mumbled something about draftees in the motor pool.

We were a logistics base where jets and helicopters were repaired and ordinance was stored. I had one enlisted man sent in by his sergeant to have his color vision checked. A note from the sergeant said he'd had to connect six color-coded wires in a helicopter to six color-coded terminals. He'd only gotten two of the six right, and if he wasn't color blind, there was going to be some serious consequences. He wasn't. There were.

We got a call from the hanger where the fighter jets were repaired. At any one time 10 percent of the fighters in the air force were at our base getting routine maintenance or repairs. These planes were equipped with ejection seats that were rated as 0-0, which meant that they were supposed to eject a pilot high enough for his parachute to open at 0 altitude and 0 air speed. They also had to kick him out of the aircraft so fast he wouldn't be split by the tail coming at him at supersonic speeds. These ejection seats had six safety pins to prevent inadvertent ejection, and any one of them would prevent firing. The mechanic working on this particular plane was repairing something under the dash, and, when he got up, apparently just reached up blindly and grabbed something to pull himself with. He grabbed the ejection lever and the rocket under the seat went off. Since the rocket would push up three hundred feet and the roof of the hanger was one hundred feet he was driven into the roof and then dropped a hundred feet to the concrete. One of my corpsmen who put him in a body bag was so upset by what he saw we had to admit him to psych and tranquilize him for a day. This was a corpsman who had served in Vietnam and thought he'd seen it all. The mechanic was a young civilian with three children, and the whole base was upset by this. We never did find out why he had all six pins removed.

There were five thousand active duty men and women on the base and twenty thousand civilians, so when it hit five in the afternoon and the colors had been lowered, there was a mad dash by the civilians to go home. I was on my way home, but when I got to the highway, there was a car that had tried to make a left turn across the highway in front of a truck and got "T-boned." When I got to the car, I found there were two passengers. They were both having agonal breathing (breathing in gasps usually occurs just before complete arrest), and since I could only try to save one by myself, I had to make a horrible choice. The driver was a young woman and had blood coming from her ear indicating a probable skull fracture and brain damage. The passenger was a ten- or eleven-year-old boy with no obvious evidence of fatal injuries. I selected the boy as most likely to revive although I noted he had an unusual appearance. The doors were sprung shut, and the seatbelt he was wearing was jammed so I started CPR with him sitting upright and me leaning in through the window. When the highway patrol arrived, they smashed out the windshield over me and managed to cut the seatbelt so we could get the kid out. The base ambulance arrived with a couple of corpsmen and we continued CPR while going to the base hospital, which was the nearest emergency facility. In our ER we got his heart restarted and started to replace fluids. Again we noted his limbs seemed very thin and he had an unusual appearance. We contacted the civilian hospital that we were bringing him and put him back in the ambulance, the highway patrol leading us into the civilian hospital. The drivers in that state seemed to ignore the sirens and lights, but the patrolman would pull up behind them and bump them in the rear bumper and that got them to move right over. The child arrested again in the ambulance, but we got him restarted and arrived at the civilian hospital with a heartbeat. I had to take the ambulance back to the scene where my car was with its four-way flashers still going, but that had used up so much of the battery that I had to get a jump from the highway patrol who was still clearing the accident scene. I asked him about the bumper bumping, and he said they had to do it all the time. Sometimes the drivers would call and complain, but the bosses simply ignored the complaints.

The civilian ER doctor called me later to tell me the boy had rearrested, and the parents had arrived to tell them the child had severe cerebral palsy. Their daughter was driving him to his physical therapy appointment when the accident happened. They jointly decided not to resuscitate him again because the additional brain damage would have left a disaster. I've always wondered if I'd chosen to try to save the girl whether things would have worked out better.

During that time Sue and I decided it was time for another baby since Doug was almost two. Sue had read an article in the magazine section of the Sunday paper about a lady in New York State who had adopted an orphan from Vietnam. This wasn't easy since there were no agencies, so all adoptions from Vietnam at that time were essentially private. Sue contacted the lady in the article and she was most helpful. She contacted the woman in the article who referred us to an orphanage in Da Nang. We contacted the sister who ran the orphanage, and we eventually agreed to adopt two children. The girl was apparently one of the sisters' favorites and would follow them around all day. The boy was just learning to stand in his crib. We began the effort of getting these adoptions through U.S. Immigration. This is the most unfriendly agency I've ever worked with, and it quickly became apparent the stock answer was no. Eventually Sue knew the regulations better than they did, and when they said no, she'd quote page and paragraph to them and they'd have to agree with her. We paid the lawyer's fees and went through another home study and got things pretty well lined up when we got a letter from the physician from the U.S. Embassy telling us that our boy was paralyzed from the waist down probably from polio. The sisters wrote and said Vinh had had a febrile illness and had quit standing in his crib. They offered us another boy, but we decided that since we'd been working for six months on getting him out, he really was ours. We couldn't leave him in Vietnam with this severe problem.

We were at the base of the Rockies and therefore got a lot of snow. I remember throwing snow nearly to the level of my head at the sides of the driveway. One day I had a man come into the ER with the story that his snow blower got jammed and he'd put it into neutral to clear the jam. He hadn't thought that with a belt drive the blades would still turn if the engine was running when there was no resistance. When he got the snow cleared, the blades began spinning and removed the tip of his index finger. Fortunately he found the tip and brought it in with him. I told him since it was cut off just at the bone we could try to reapply the tip, which I did. Fortunately it took as a graft without any complications. He was so grateful to have his finger back he brought me a lovely bottle of Scotch. People never seem to be able to keep their fingers out of places they shouldn't be. One lady came with the story that she'd had her Osterizer jam and had put her finger in to clear the jam, which unfortunately she did. She wanted to know if I could fix her finger, but I had to explain I couldn't make a finger out of hamburger, so she ended up with a partial amputation.

Since I was the only one with advanced training, I was the backup for complicated OB and Internal Medicine when the specialists were out of town or otherwise unavailable. One day I got an OB stat page and on arrival found the junior OB sitting at the delivery table with one child in a bassinet and a small hand hanging out the mother's vagina. This was the days before ultrasound and they had not realized there were twins. You cannot deliver a shoulder presentation and we didn't have rapid C-section capabilities so I had to do a procedure called a version extraction. I'd read about these and knew what to do, but I'd never had to do it before. You put on a special glove that comes nearly to your shoulder and reach inside the uterus to find the feet. You then turn the fetus from shoulder to feet first and do a breech extraction. Although scary, the procedure went fine, and we delivered a second girl with both babies about five pounds. I was very concerned that we didn't have the facilities to take care of a sick baby, so I called the nearby university hospital neonatal unit to transfer them, but they told me their transfer incubators were tied up and they couldn't come to get them. I had the corpsman warm up one of the cosmopolitans as hot as the heater would go and put the babies in bassinets with oxygen running and transported them myself. Believe me it was plenty warm in there. They did fine and returned in a few days. They had had a placental steal (one baby getting more of the blood than the other), so the nurses had nicknamed them Rose Red and Snow White because of their complexions.

I had one elderly couple come in complaining of tiredness, which is one of those dreaded complaints physicians fear. Frequently you fail to find any reason, and often this is psychological, but sometimes it's a serious physical problem. I ran the usual tests on the couple and discovered they both had very low potassium levels. There are several sources of this, most frequently drugs, but try as I might, I couldn't find what was causing this. I could raise their levels with supplemental potassium but they would go right back to their previous levels in a couple of weeks. I asked our Internal Medicine specialist to look at them for me but he had no greater luck than I had and he sent them back to me. One day they were in, and in our conversation the old man said his jaw hurt. I asked him why, and he said he thought it was from the licorice he was chewing. My ears immediately perked up, and I asked how much licorice he was eating. He told me they had both had problems with constipation and had read that licorice would help with that. They were each eating about half pound of licorice daily and had been for months. The older literature reports that licorice caused low potassium, but this is so rare today both the Internist and I had failed to ask about it. The small amounts most people eat of this substance wouldn't do this, but the huge amounts this couple was taking in certainly would. We found a better way to correct their constipation, and their potassium took care of itself when they stopped the licorice. I ask about it now but that's the only time I've seen it in a lifetime of medicine. It showed me that sometimes just talking with your patient will cause the answer to pop up.

There is a thing in the air force called TDY, which stands for a temporary duty assignment, and a lot of personnel are assigned to go on these usually for a class but for many other reasons as well. I quickly learned there were two groups of guys. One group would come in to get a penicillin shot even if they didn't have symptoms of an STD (sexually transmitted disease), and the other group would have symptoms of prostatitis, which can be from an STD but more often seemed due to disuse.

STDs were always a problem when you had five thousand troops (mostly men) on the base, but one young airman stood out above the others. He had just gotten into the air force and probably was away from home for the first time. He came in on sick call with gonorrhea twice in a two-week period, and when I suggested if he kept this up we'd put the penicillin in the offending organ, he returned with crab lice. I explained to him I could treat this with two methods. One, we could use a shampoo with insecticide in it, or two, we could shave the area where crabs lived (the pubis). The insecticide was dangerous if used too much, so I was going to use it once but if he returned I would have my sergeant shave him. That finally got through and I didn't see him back.

Our active duty people weren't always very medically literate, and I had one sergeant come back after being given suppositories for his hemorrhoids complaining that those chewy pills he'd been given didn't work. I rewrote his prescription and substituted the word "rectum" with "ass," and then he understood what to do with them. One active duty person came wanting a refill on his placebos (pills without medication), which were clearly labeled on his bottle, so I told him we might not have the same brand but we had the same medicine even if it came in another color. He was very relieved and told me it was the only medicine he'd had that worked for him.

Since we were in a sportsmen's paradise I decided to go deer hunting. I went with a couple of our sergeants and got a nice deer. When we got ready to leave, the entire back of his vehicle was filled with deer.

I asked him how he had enough tags, and he told me he had other people on base buy tags and then he filled them and brought them the meat. I ended having to ride back sitting on top of a pile of dead deer.

One day a master sergeant came in on sick call and told me he'd just come back from a tour in Vietnam and was having trouble adjusting to the food; since getting back, he was always constipated. His abdomen seemed somewhat bloated, but with the beer belly he had, it was a little hard to tell. I put him on some stool softeners and high bulk agents and told him to push water and to return in a few days if this didn't work. He did return in three days saying he'd been unable to have a bowel movement and he was definitely bloated with his abdomen sounding like a drum. This time I did a rectal to see if he was impacted with stool, but instead I found a rock solid tumor with my finger. I sent him over to the surgeon but his lab work showed the liver was involved and any surgery was just going to provide relief. I suspected he only had a few months at most. How ironic he'd gotten back from Vietnam fine. I did wonder if he'd had a rectal exam as part of his physical before going overseas.

One morning I came in to find my two desk sergeants laughing about the night before. It seems the pediatrician was MOD and was working in the ER when a young second lieutenant right out of the academy came and wanted to throw his almost nonexistent weight around. He started harassing my desk sergeants about why he had to wait his turn. The hospital had a policy that rank had nothing to do with when you were seen. You would be moved up the list if you were in dire trouble, but otherwise it was first come, first served. The sergeants were trying to explain this to this young man when they saw the pediatrician walk past and go down to his call room. They told me they were pretty upset with the doc until he came back down the hall in full uniform with his major's leaves clearly visible. He put the smart aleck at attention in front of the whole waiting room and made him stand there until his wing-commander came in and got him. Needless to say, his CO wasn't happy to give up his evening to come get his bad boy.

We were encouraged to go to medical conferences, and I elected to go to one being held at Park City, Utah. Most of the attendees would go to the lectures, which started at 6:00 a.m., and then go skiing for the afternoon. There were classes for those who didn't want to go, and since I didn't know how to ski, I stayed for the classes. One of the classes was by a former surgeon who had become a psychiatrist and who used a lot of hypnosis in his practice. We were taught induction techniques and what we could and couldn't do with hypnosis. Afterward I included it in my practice. Since hypnosis would take more time than was allotted for an appointment, I would schedule this last in the day.

One woman had stress headaches, which were very resistant to treatment, so I thought I'd try hypnotherapy with her. When I first induced her, she changed her voice and mannerisms, and on a whim I asked her name and she gave me a different name than she had used when she came in. I was totally startled but proceeded to question her and learned that this personality was aware there were two of them in this one person and could come and go as she wished. The usual public personality was unaware of this but did tell me that sometimes she found herself in circumstances she couldn't explain like waking in a motel room with a man and not remembering how she'd gotten there. I talked with the base psychiatrist about her, but he said this was so rare he didn't know any more about it than I did, so I went ahead and worked with her. Eventually we got her to one personality and her headaches stopped (remember we were draining the swamp?).

One of my GMOs had to have his wisdom teeth extracted, and he told me he was terrified of needles. He asked if I would hypnotize him for the pain. I talked with the dentist who was going to do the procedure, and he was a little reluctant but agreed to try if he could anesthetize one side. We agreed this would be a good test so I induced the doc several times to get him used to the procedure, and we went ahead. I induced him and suggested he could feel no pain in his mouth, and the dentist went ahead and used his needle on the one side without discomfort. The teeth were removed but the root of one went into the maxillary sinus. This occurred on the side, which had no chemical anesthetic but the dentist was able to repair it entirely under hypnosis. What really surprised me was that I was able to suggest he would have no post-op pain or swelling, and indeed my GMO was back at work the next day.

One wife of an active duty NCO who was overseas came in with a minor complaint, but I noticed something strange in the way she looked at me. She seemed to stare intently at me in a very unusual way. At first I was suspicious that, with her seeming flat affect (minimal emotional response to what's happening), she was schizophrenic but she seemed to be normal in other ways. I talked to her about what she did with herself all day, and apparently since her husband was gone she watched TV a lot. While we were talking, I covered my mouth, and suddenly she couldn't understand what I was saying. She had apparently had a gradual hearing loss, and without realizing it had learned lip reading from her TV shows. We got her an appointment at our consulting base in California where they had an ENT and I didn't see her again.

One day I was called to the ER because they had scrambled an ambulance for a report of "man down" in front of the officer's club, which was only a couple blocks from the hospital. The corpsmen sent out reported they had an officer in an unusual uniform who was in complete arrest. They started CPR and raced back to the ER where we were setting up. They had barely pulled in when a half dozen staff cars pulled in behind them with the base commanding officer and other big wigs. My chief nurse threw them out of the ER and made them wait outside. Rank didn't buy you anything when we had an emergency. After trying to revive the man for a reasonable period of time, I had to call the code off and pronounce him dead. It turned out he was second in command of the British Royal Air Force and was attending a meeting on our base. He'd just had a large fancy lunch at the Officers' Club and was walking back to the meeting. I was very irritated with the Brits when I found he had a known ventricular aneurysm (a weak place in the wall of the heart, which was ballooning out), and they hadn't warned us they were sending a man with such a severe heart condition to our base.

Since we were a small hospital with very limited staff, we had to rely on the Medevac system a lot. These are a number of aircraft around the country who have hospital facilities aboard and transport sick and not-so-sick patients from one base to another. Only one of them was equipped with sea-level pressure, and the others used the cabin pressure system of the commercial airlines, which is a percentage of the outside pressure usually something below six thousand feet. We had one patient who needed an immediate heart valve replacement and was barely surviving at our base, which was at five thousand feet. When we called for immediate Medevac to Brooks Army Hospital where they had a team that could do heart valves, we found the only plane available was not the sea-level plane. I reasoned that if he could survive at our altitude, we could get by if the pilot didn't go higher in his cabin pressure. He wasn't happy about it but agreed to follow the highways through the mountain passes, which would keep him below ten thousand feet and keep the cabin pressure at safe levels. The patient got to Brooks just fine.

Another patient we Medevac'd out was a patient with a chronic productive cough and fever who was very short of breath. I'd talked with the pulmonologist at Brooks about him, and he felt the man probably had a fungal lung infection but we couldn't rule out TB. We didn't think we had the six weeks it would take to rule TB out with cultures (TB grows very slowly in culture), so we agreed to put a mask on him and tell Medevac he didn't have TB so they would transport him. It turned he did indeed have aspergilosis, which is what we suspected all along.

Before we had a psychiatrist on base I had a sergeant who had just recently returned from the Philippines, which he hated. He'd made the mistake of marrying the ex-wife of a high-ranking officer. She would go to the Officers' Club and party with her friends. He, of course, wasn't allowed into the Officers' Club. This became such a point of contention that they got into a fight and he hit her and ended up chasing her down the street with her naked. She arrived at the base commander's office the next day with a black eye. The commander immediately ordered the sergeant back to the Philippines. I had already been seeing him for his problems and had diagnosed him as having a situational depression, so when he came to me for help, I called his wing commander who also thought the woman had a lot to do with the circumstance. He asked me if the man had a psychiatric diagnosis and I told him he did. The wing commander informed me that it was against regulations to send air force personnel overseas with an active psychiatric diagnosis. He also told me he would be happy to transfer the man in the States but couldn't for another six weeks because he'd only recently gotten back. I admitted the man with the psychiatric diagnosis and he sat in the hospital. Shortly I got an inquiry from the general's office wanting to transfer the man to the Philippines, and I told them what the wing commander had told me. The general wanted to order me to rescind the diagnosis, but I had read the regulations regarding psychiatric diagnosis and told him I couldn't remove the diagnosis. Although I could make the diagnosis it could only be removed by a psychiatrist, which we didn't have. I told him we'd arrange for the patient to be Medevac'd to the consulting base where there was a psychiatrist. After a couple weeks I got a very upset colonel in my office wanting to know why the man hadn't gone to the consulting base. I pointed out that Medevac had priorities, and this man was classified a four, which meant they would take him if they were in our area but would not make a special trip. The colonel offered me the general's personal plane, but I had to refuse because I could only use Medevac for a patient, by regulation. My boss had been out of town, but on his return, I got a call about what had I been doing to upset the general. I told him the situation and that in a few days we'd been informed the medevac would arrive to take the patient to the consultant. That is indeed what happened, and a few days later I got a call from the consulting psychiatrist asking if the patient was being screwed as it appeared. I assured him he was. He said not to worry about it because he was going to send the patient back, but he'd keep the chart in his desk until I called him and told him the patient had been transferred inside the States for which he would be eligible in a short time. When the patient got back the general immediately wanted him sent to the Philippines but I had to tell him we hadn't gotten the chart back so couldn't certify that the diagnosis had been lifted. A few days later his wing commander transferred him inside the States, and amazingly enough his chart turned up right after he'd cleared base. Using medical regulations, we had managed to save the sergeant from the manipulations of the general.

The pressures on the enlisted men were sometimes quite considerable. I had a tech sergeant I found kneeling on the floor of a storage room and clutching his chest. He told me he was having severe chest pain and was afraid he was having a heart attack. We admitted him to our ICU and went through all the motions but could find no organic source for his discomfort. I finally got him to talk with me and found he hadn't been able to get home in the previous seven years and was just trying to hold on until his retirement came up the next year. He admitted having anxiety attacks, and we decided to send him to our consulting base to see the psychiatrist. He was medevaced but returned in a few days and told me they had admitted him to the psych ward. He said after the first two patients he met both told him they were Jesus Christ; he decided he'd better straighten up because that place wasn't for him. I was able to get him a compassionate transfer to a base near his home and hope he was able to get his retirement.

In those days homosexuals weren't allowed to serve in the armed forces. I had one rather frail young man walk into my office with the tube we carried from base to base with our pay records still under his arm from basic. He had never actually signed into base. He told me his recruiting officer knew he was gay but told him that would be no problem. It appeared recruiting officers would say anything to fulfill their quotas. We had specific orders about homosexuality and I had to send him along to the office that oversaw his discharge and return home. Unfortunately he now had a general discharge on his record, which could be a negative on his chances for a job.

Our people came from all over, and one night in mid-winter when it was below zero and the wind was blowing near forty miles per hour, a young airman was sent in from the flight line where they get planes ready. He was from Puerto Rico and had just returned from a year in Vietnam. He'd never been in cold weather, let alone the kind of arctic conditions we were having. He was shivering and appeared somewhat blue. I determined he was just suffering from hypothermia, and we kept him in the ER until we got him warmed up. He appeared to have all the recommended cold weather gear, but it was nowhere near enough for this lad. I had to tell him he was going to be returned to duty, but it was near dawn and maybe things would warm up somewhat. He told me if he was forced to work in such conditions, he would go AWOL. I explained to him the consequences of such an action and suggested he talk to his sergeant about his cold intolerance. I never saw him again, so I don't know what he decided.

Our people not only came from all over the country, they came from all sorts of environments. One day in early fall we were told there were two airmen missing in the mountains. These were city boys who had decided to try their hands at hunting. Enlisted personnel could rent hunting guns on base, and they had done so. They had no real knowledge of the mountains, so they went with light jackets and combat boots out into the mountains. When they didn't return, their car was found by the road, and the local sheriff's rescue people went looking. Their technique was interesting in that they went outward from the point of origin in straight lines and built fires just in sight of each other. The idea was that either they would find the men or the men would cross one of the lines, see the fires and follow them either to the base or to the person setting the fires. It worked and they were brought into the hospital with hypothermia and frostbitten feet. We had thought we would be forced to amputate, but their injuries eventually demarcated at the toes, so they only lost some toes but probably had chilblains (excessive reaction to cold with a lot of pain) for several years.

Sometimes a patient with MS will get a form of euphoria. I had one such patient who was very funny even though she had a bad disease. She had an amazing southern accent and would frequently come up with expressions like "I don't want to be the crabgrass on the lawn of your life." She became even crazier when I had to hospitalize her to use very high dose steroids on her disease and to be able to send her to private PT where she was getting ice whirlpool to decrease the muscle spasms. She became very flirty, and we had to tell the corpsmen to leave her care to the nurses. She liked to sit Indian fashion on the bed wearing baby doll tops and no bottoms and call out to the young corpsmen asking for something or other. Fortunately she seemed to respond to the therapy, and we were able to taper the medication and get her out in a relatively short time.

Being in the military, we naturally had frequent disaster drills, but one day the fire and rescue had a drill going when we got a call from the tower that they had an in-flight emergency. We were not aware of the drill being done by the fire people but since wewere on the same radio net, things got very confused, because they were simulating a fire on a train on base while we were responding to the in-flight emergency. It wasn't clear whether we should roll more than one crash wagon or not, but I finally got the on-scene commander on the radio and got things cleared up. He had to pull some of his people from the practice drill to respond to the real thing at the runway.

Rank in the military creates problems for the medical personnel. The career military couldn't understand that a hospital has one rank and that may not correspond to the military rank. Our chief nurse was a lieutenant colonel, but she was old school and she and her nurses would stand when a physician came on the ward and offer him their seats.

The higher-ranking officers would expect special treatment, and they sometimes got it in ways they hadn't planned. I came in one morning and found one of my senior corpsmen sewing up a full colonel who was yelling and complaining constantly. When I looked on the tray the corpsman was using, there was no anesthetic, only saline (salt water). The corpsman was grinning from ear to ear. I just passed by and asked the corpsmen at the desk what was up, and they told me the colonel had been nasty and throwing his weight around from the moment he had come in. I decided just to act like I knew nothing. Another time my nurse came to my office and said, "You'd better get down there or they're going to kill him." The "him" she was referring to was a full colonel who had a splinter in his finger. The corpsman had a tray out with a knife on it but again no anesthetic. I told him to go on and I'd take care of the colonel. After numbing him with local, I removed the large splinter easily and got the story that he was building a cabin in the mountains, had gotten the splinter but couldn't get it out himself, and had to drive a long distance back to base to get it removed. Naturally he was upset by the time he got back and had been taking it out on my corpsmen. I explained to him it was a very foolish response to pick on people who were authorized to cut on you.

We had a training unit on the base for parajumpers. These guys were the very epitome of being gung-ho and even ran from class to class in formation and yelling in cadence. We had two of them who were brought in because their parachutes wouldn't open. One of them told me he managed to get his reserve chute deployed but only at the last minute, and since it was attached to his belly, it just had time to jerk him, so he landed flat on his back. The second one never got anything to open but sky dived to get maximum wind resistance and apparently landed on his feet and rolled since both ankles were broken as were numerous other bones. The amazing thing was that one of them couldn't wait to get out of the ICU so he could go back to jumping. We had to explain that with a couple collapsed vertebrae in his back, it wasn't feasible to release him back to jumping.

Secrecy is always present on military bases and ours was no exception. I had one man from a top-secret unit come in with a problem with his back. When I asked if he was required to lift more than ten pounds as part of his job, he said that was classified. I explained that I wasn't interested in what he lifted only whether he had to lift, but he still refused to answer so I had to write an excuse without knowing whether it was appropriate or not.

One section of our base was full of bunkers, which stored bombs and other ordinance and was very carefully monitored; a second section was simply off limits. One of the flight surgeons and I were bow hunters, and there was a bow-hunting range on the ordinance portion of the base where you could walk and find various targets along the path. We went out one day to try this out, but we got lost and found ourselves driving around on little roads surrounded by numerous bunkers. After a little way we noticed we were being followed by a jeep with two air police. They didn't try to stop us, probably because he was a captain and I was a major, but they made us so nervous we finally found an exit from that area and simply left. We never did get to go to the range.

One Saturday I was MOD when a young man in civvies came in with a man with credentials of a local police detective and a sobbing woman. The young man approached the desk and said he wanted the woman to undergo a rape exam. He identified himself as working for OIS but claimed his rank was classified. I asked where the alleged rape had occurred, and he named a subdivision just off base. I had to explain we were prohibited by regulation from doing such an exam unless the crime had occurred on base because we would then be subject to civilian subpoenas. He said he was ordering me to do the exam, and I told him that wasn't going to happen. He then wanted to talk to the hospital commander, and I explained I was the commander since the colonel was out of town and I was MOD. I told him I did know the colonel who commanded the OIS on base, and I would call him if the young man didn't get out of my ER. The civilian detective had been trying to get him to go to a private hospital as the evidence was aging so they finally left. I'm reasonably sure that young man had a rank no higher than sergeant and was just trying to show off for the civilian.

The JAG (Judge Advocate General's) office on base was run by a full colonel who had been in for many years (he'd actually been a paratrooper during Normandy), and he was rather corpulent. He'd gone skiing and was bragging to a friend of his while standing in the lift line about how he'd been able to avoid the weight requirements the air force had. Unfortunately for him the next person in the line was one of our flight surgeons. When the colonel got back to base, he found orders to report to the flight surgeon's office first thing in the morning.

This same man retired while at our base and his retirement party was fantastic. He knew people all over the air force, and they sent food from whatever area they were in. This all came in on courier plane and included such things as fresh Maine lobsters. I wished I was invited but no such luck.

As I neared the end of my military obligation, I began to think about what I wanted to do in private practice. I had already turned down an offer to take over a practice in the central valley of California. The physician was very busy but his practice included a lot of things I ethically couldn't do, such as giving B12 shots to old ladies to make them feel better, basically as a placebo. I arranged enough leave to travel up and down the West Coast because we had decided we'd like to get back near the ocean. We decided we didn't want to go to Southern California again but over time saw nearly every town north of San Francisco. I went to a meeting of the AAFP in San Francisco and found a note on a bulletin board there saying a town on the coast needed primary care badly and was building a new hospital, so we drove north after the conference to look at what was available.

We found another town with a brand-new hospital, which was recruiting, but I quickly learned the older physicians in the area were unhappy with the new hospital and really the hospital was recruiting to get physicians who would refer to them. I didn't want to start practice in a town with a turf battle going on so we moved on.

We found a very nice but very small town that wanted new physicians and were shown around by a physician who worked at the small local hospital doubling both as the pathologist and the anesthesiologist. He was very nice, but when Sue asked what they did at night there, he said they went down to the highway and watched the trucks go by. *Bad answer*. My wife immediately wrote them off, and when I found the three primary care physicians in town were all over seventy and just waiting for new blood so they could retire, I could see that I would be killed with too many patients and I too wrote them off.

When we got to the town that had advertised, we found they were about ten miles from a larger town and had a small university so that answered what there was to do. The old hospital was a creaky old frame structure, but when we arrived, a number of the physicians met with us in a coffee room and welcomed us to the community. We were then shown the place where the footings for the new hospital were dug and the new office building next door was in the same stage of construction. This was eventually to be our choice, but we did continue north into Oregon and found a town I would have liked except when I talked to several physicians they had stories of a turf war between the specialists and the primary care physicians. Again not a place I wanted to be to start out.

Once we'd tentatively settled on our new town, I began to look toward what it would take to open an office. I called to get a phone number reserved, and the lady taking the order asked for an appointment, saying she'd lived in the area for six months and hadn't been able to get a physician. I began to list the equipment I'd need and placed an ad in the local paper for office assistants. I got a number of good applicants, including a young woman with only one arm and no legs. This lady was hired by a new internist before I could interview her, but she subsequently became a good friend and had an effect on our lives later.

I knew absolutely nothing about business, so I got a book from a company called Medical Economics and that was my business course.

They recommended such things as using a bookkeeping method you understood and that proved crucial. I often felt, however, that it would have been cheaper to get an MBA than to learn business the way I did.

I took another quick trip back to find a house and interview applicants for office staff. I found an old house with four or more bedrooms (we'd been notified the kids were coming from Vietnam soon). It was a mess and had been a hippy commune. It did have a neat indoor pool, and I thought I would be able to fix it up. I consulted with Sue and we decided to buy it. I hired a handyman to shovel out the rugs and trash and clean it up for us.

I hired two excellent office assistants, one more a clerk who had been with NASA arranging astronaut physicals and the other a back office person who had experience as an ECG tech and a lab assistant as well as a back office assistant. I began to get a feel for some things going on in town as well. Both the women I hired had applied at another new office and refused to continue to interview there when the doctor insisted they have a complete physical done *by him.* I'm going to call the doc "Sam" and will talk about him in detail later.

When we finally moved we gave our old Buick Skylark to the fellows who cleaned our house for us because it wouldn't cross the desert again. Fortunately the air force was packing and moving us, and off we went to California.

Solo Practice

When we arrived in our new home, Sue began setting up the house and preparing for the arrival of the kids while I was extremely busy getting the office under way. I had a bank loan gotten solely on my signature (this town was desperate for docs). I had hired my office staff, and we began ordering exam tables and equipment as well as setting up the front office with the record files and bookkeeping files. I bought a new station wagon without much negotiation just because I was in a big hurry getting the office set up.

We opened the office the day after Labor Day and had a full book of appointments from day one, based on an announcement in the local paper. My first patient was a woman I would come to know very well over the years as she worked in the hospital. Her complaints were very strange, and I'm not sure I would have worked it out if she hadn't had a letter from the U.S. Forrest Service telling her that they were aware of several cases of relapsing fever from a camp ground she'd stayed in that summer in Colorado. I excused myself for a moment and ran into my office to look this up. It turned out to be a tick-born disease caused by an organism related to the one that caused syphilis. I began to wonder if this was private practice, would I be able to handle it? The lab tests failed to confirm the disease, but they frequently did fail, and the symptoms were perfect so I went ahead and treated her. Sometimes there's a reaction to treatment and she had that reaction, which pretty much confirmed the diagnosis.

That first day was chaos as we didn't have our procedures down, and we didn't know where things were because we'd just stuck them in cabinets as they'd arrived. As a result we didn't get done until about seven thirty and we were all three worn out. Fortunately the ladies were troopers, and we were able to all work together. Each evening we got closer to our expected closing time. I took the day's receipts to the night drop at the bank each evening on my way home and noticed one of the older docs in town, whose office was next to the bank, was always still working, so I didn't feel so bad. He didn't have appointments and just saw everyone who came in. This technique is being advocated again today. If we don't remember past mistakes, we get to repeat them.

One of my major expenses was malpractice insurance because I did complicated OB and did C-sections. When a seventeen-year-old girl at term walked into the office requesting obstetrical care and I found out she'd had no prenatal care at all, I wasn't very happy. I could see my medical career going down the tubes after less than a week of practice. We pointed out to her that it was required to pay for OB care in advance, and it would cost $700. Her father had accompanied her, and he asked us to wait and ran out and drove away in a beat-up old pickup truck. A few minutes later he returned with an old mason jar full of money and still dripping dirt from being dug up. He opened it and counted out the money and I was *stuck*. Upon examining the girl, I found she was in early labor, so I called over to the hospital to get her admitted but they told me they were completely full and had no bed for her. I contacted the county hospital in the next town, and they could take her but my privileges hadn't cleared the committees there so the on-call OB would have to take her. I gave the family their money back and heaved a sigh of relief as they drove off.

Just after we opened the office the kids began to arrive from Vietnam. Vinh first and Thanh three months later. We knew he had been sick so rather than try to keep him in a motel overnight, we chartered a small plane, which didn't cost much more than a commercial flight. We arranged for the pilot to wait while we got him and she flew us home that night. He had had chickenpox and was covered with secondarily infected pox. He also was paralyzed from the waist down and got around by dragging himself with his arms, so I got his infections cleared up, and we started him in physical therapy.

When Thanh arrived she was accompanied by Americans returning to the States. One of the men brought her off the plane and it turned out that for whatever reason she had decided she didn't want anything to do with women. Sue was very disappointed, but she came to me easily, and we were able to stay in a motel at the airport and fly home the next morning. We'd been told she had a scalp infection, but she looked fine in the little cap she was wearing. When we took the cap off she looked like a little monk with a tonsure with the whole top of her head bald with ringworm. Shortly after we got home I had her on medication and her head cleared up rapidly. She made a 180-degree change and would only go to Sue and screamed if I tried to pick her up. At this point we had three in diapers and the washing machine was running constantly until the transmission broke (I didn't even know they had one).

The office next to mine housed a pair of GPs who were husband and wife. They were good docs and had two very nice, if active, little boys. One day the father was telling me he had a family who had such poor hygiene their kids had come in with scabies. This is a skin mite that is microscopic in size and burrows into the skin, causing a nasty itchy allergic reaction. Although the Romans knew how to treat it, the treatment was forgotten in the middle ages when it was referred to as the seven-year itch. I told him I didn't think it was really a hygiene problem, but he was convinced it was. A few weeks later his wife brought their kids in because of an itchy rash, and I got to tease him about his family's hygiene.

Adjusting to a new hospital and its staff is difficult, and I had to learn what their ways were and what I could accept and what I couldn't. I had a patient who came in with chest pain and the ECG showed he was having a heart attack. I admitted him to the ICU-CCU and started standard regimens. I thought to be safe I'd get an internal medicine consult. There was one internist at that time who apparently had ruled the roost with the GPs not willing to challenge him. I sent the consult request, and the next day when I made rounds, I found my patient was no longer in the CCU but had been transferred to the general floor and a whole new set of orders written. The nurses told me the internist had done this. I talked to the patient and asked him if he was firing me, and he said no, so I had to write orders that unless the patient fired me, I *was the doc of record and other docs were not to write orders.* I had a discussion with the internist about the difference between a consult (give me your opinion about management) and a referral (please take over the case). I created a consult/referral form for use in the future, and it was passed by the staff, which allowed the GPs to get out from under the internist's thumb.

Another requirement of privileges for surgery is that the new doctor must be monitored by a staff physician. Since none of the staff did C-sections, they assigned a general surgeon to monitor me. He was a devout Catholic. He would help me do C-sections, and then if the patient had requested a postpartum tubal ligation, he would go stand in the corner facing away from the table while the scrub nurse and I tied the tubes. After that was done, he would come back and assist me in closing.

One patient came to the office complaining that his "hemorrhoids" were killing him. He'd been to see a couple of other docs without relief from the creams they'd prescribed and wanted to know what else could be done. When I examined him, I found a hard mass protruding from his rectum. He told me none of the other physicians had even looked. I had to explain to him this had nothing to do with his hemorrhoids. I put in some local anesthetic and did a biopsy, which came back as a cloacal carcinoma, which is a very rare cancer from a fetal tissue remnant and generally has a poor prognosis. I sent him out for oncological treatment, but eventually he died of his tumor. I always wondered if he would have done better if the previous docs had just done the somewhat unpleasant exam they should have done. Cutting corners is usually a lousy idea in medicine.

One of my patients told me he was staying young by going to Mexico to a "rejuvenation" clinic. There they would (for considerable money) give him lamb's placenta by IV. He was quite convinced this was going to keep him young, and although I did express doubts, there really was no point in getting into a fight with him. He'd already been warned by the "doctors" in Mexico that this wasn't known to American doctors, and they would be jealous of such advanced techniques. Since he would have immediately died of anaphylaxis if he'd been given such an infusion, I was sure he was only getting IV fluids and just left it at that. It made him feel better psychologically anyway.

One day the scheduler asked if I would see a lady in place of her husband who had originally made the appointment. She was complaining of a severe headache for several days. She wasn't totally coherent, and when I asked her husband about drug usage, he said she'd taken about a hundred Darvons over the past two days. Since this drug is related to opiates, in some respects it certainly could cause confusion, so I asked him to take the drugs away from her and come back the next day so I could assess her mental status. The next morning they arrived and she was no different, so I took her to the hospital and did a spinal tap, which showed red cells that were several days old indicating a bleed. Angiography showed an aneurysm, which was almost certainly the source. The neurosurgeon in the next town told me that 50 percent of these cases died at the time of the bleed and the rest would have about two weeks before they would bleed again. The presence of the blood made the vessels in the area prone to spasm, so he wanted to wait ten days to let things settle down. They put her in the ICU at his hospital, but at four days, she began to have worse symptoms, and a repeat angiogram showed she was having a new bleed so he took her to surgery. Unfortunately I couldn't help him as I was literally going to the airport to fly to San Francisco to take my board exam. When I got back, I learned she had died. I also learned she'd gotten the Darvon from her physician father who was a neurosurgeon. When he talked to me on the phone, he said we'd handled the situation exactly right, and it was just the luck of the draw. A couple weeks later her husband again returned, this time for his original appointment, and when I looked at him as a patient rather than a spouse of a patient, I realized he had the most protuberant eyes I'd seen in a long time. That coupled with his story of nervousness and weight loss confirmed the diagnosis of hyperthyroidism so I got him on suppressive medication and scheduled him with a local surgeon who had experience in thyroidectomy. It was a little humbling to realize that such a blatant diagnosis could be right in front of me, and since I wasn't thinking of the person as a patient, I'd missed it entirely.

One man came to me complaining of pain in the pelvis or low abdomen. The exam showed a rock-hard prostate, and the x-ray showed lesions in the pelvic bones. It was apparent that he had prostatic carcinoma even though he was only in his fifties. Prostatic cancer is quite variable in its virulence, but when the patient is as young as this, it tends to be very rapidly advancing. There were a pair of older urologists in the next town, and I called one of them and told him the story and asked if he would do a biopsy. He said he didn't need a biopsy and that the man was going to die soon and essentially hung up on me. There was a new doc in our town who, although not trained specifically as an oncologist, had worked in an oncology office in Southern California. He agreed to start chemotherapy if we had biopsy proof of prostate cancer. Unfortunately chemo had never been especially effective with this cancer. I ended up reading on the procedure of prostate biopsy, and I was very familiar with the needles used because they were also used in liver biopsy. I went ahead and did the biopsy, and of course it was primary prostatic cancer, so we started him on a chemotherapy regimen, which did seem to help for a while, but eventually the cancer escaped the effects of the drugs and the patient died about two years later.

We frequently had problems with the specialists in the next town because they were very busy, and they were in the habit of riding roughshod over the docs in our town. They very much resented the fact that we were recruiting docs in their specialties. One day I was seeing a patient of mine in the ER, which was very busy, and was just sitting at the desk waiting on lab results when the radio squawked to life with a call from the ambulance saying they were en route with a patient who seemed to have a broken leg. Almost immediately after that, the phone rang. Since the ER personnel were all busy, I answered it by saying "ER" at which time the person on the other end identified himself as an orthopedic surgeon in the next town who was notorious for screaming at staff. He didn't know who I was and started shouting at me with multiple curse words to the effect that the person in the ambulance was his patient, and he didn't want the new orthopedic surgeon in our town to "steal his patient." After listening for a few seconds, I decided I didn't have to listen to that so I simply hung up. When he arrived at the ER, he wanted to know who the h—had hung up on him. I introduced myself as a new primary care specialist in the area, and he suddenly became very apologetic. I guess he didn't want to irritate a possible source of referrals.

I had a run of patients with bowel problems who all had a rock hard mass when I did a rectal exam. I had to take them to the ER to do the biopsy through the proctoscope because I didn't have one yet. It reached the point I was afraid to do that exam for fear of what I would find. After four in a row, it let off, but of the four patients only one had a chance because the other three cancers were already through the mucosa and chemo therapy just didn't work once that cancer had spread. We had to operate on all of them to remove the large mass and get pathological exams of the mucosa, but none of them lasted very long.

With a busy practice and especially with lots of kids in the practice, I got phone calls 24/7. It seemed like it would never let up, to the point that Sue and I went down the road about sixty miles and took a motel room for the weekend just to get some peace and quiet. I had another doc who agreed to cover for me while I was out of town, but he wasn't interested in any call-sharing arrangement as a regular thing, and he'd send patients to the ER, which was employing anyone with a license. Some of them were pretty bad.

While I was gone, one of my patients, a forty-five-year-old man, went to the ER with a temperature of 104 and shortness of breath. The ER "physician" heard rales (the sound of fluid in the air sacks of the lungs), diagnosed congestive heart failure, and gave the patient a diuretic. When I saw the man Monday, it was obvious even to a layman he had pneumonia, and I put him on the appropriate antibiotic. This so-called doc could easily have killed the patient. That left me no choice but to see all my own patients when they showed up at the ER.

One of the things we were trained in in a Family Medicine residency was counseling and I had one of my more difficult cases turn up early in my practice. A woman had come in for initial OB care and asked about marriage counseling as well. I asked her what the problems were, and she explained the baby wasn't her husband's. I explained that marriage counseling wasn't intended to "save" a marriage but to explore what would be the best resolution. She said she wanted to continue the marriage, and she thought her husband did too. We arranged joint visits and worked with the couple for several months. In the end they resolved to stay together, and he accepted the new baby as his own although, because the biological father was Native American, the child looked nothing like her blond father. I took care of that child for many years. She and her blond sister got along great, and as far as I could tell, the father treated them both the same.

One woman came in for vaginal bleeding and told me the strange story that she had "passed something" on the bank of a river in the nearby mountains. When I examined her, it was pretty apparent she'd delivered a baby size "something," and when asked about this, she just acted dumb. I admitted her for the bleeding and took her to the OR to repair the tears and to do a D and C to get tissue to ensure she hadn't passed a choriocarcinoma (a cancer of the placenta, which grows on its own with the pregnancy dying early). I felt that there appeared to be a baby left on the stream bank, and I was obligated to report the situation to the sheriff's department. They were decidedly uninterested. First they pointed out that the river was on the boundary with another county and therefore might not be in their jurisdiction. They did send out an investigator to talk to me, but he decided that there were bears in that area so it was a waste of time to have anyone go look. I discharged the lady the next day. I still think she left a baby out to die.

OB at the hospital was still in the dark ages. They had no monitors, and most deliveries were done with no anesthesia except local. I had been lobbying for monitors but to no avail until I found an article about a hospital in Puerto Rico where they lost a case based on not having monitors. The court ruled if they could not afford modern equipment, they shouldn't be practicing OB. I took the article to the hospital administrator, and he got so upset he refused to let the Coriometrics (a monitor manufacturer) rep. who was there demonstrating the monitors to remove the demo until a new one was delivered.

We had a large population of hippies who had moved to our area from San Francisco and who wanted to live "naturally." When I arrived, I asked OB to get some epidural kits in but I never was able to use them as the women were all Lamaze trained and didn't want anything else. One of the problems that arose was a desire for home deliveries, which was partially met by two lay midwives who were very careful and the "Peoples School of Medicine" who weren't. This group was led by a young man who wore full-length white robes and a full beard (very obviously trying to look like Jesus) and whose sole credentials consisted of having been an army corpsman. They had a van that they took to the delivery and parked on the street. The local law enforcement knew they were acting illegally but couldn't get enough evidence.

One day I was called to the ER as backup OB to see a young lady with a placenta that had not delivered after she had been delivered of her baby. This can cause severe bleeding as it prevents the uterus from cramping down and closing off the vessels. When I examined her, I found she had had an episiotomy (a cut in the vaginal tissue to make more room for the baby's head). The local women wouldn't tell you how this occurred, but this girl was from out of town and readily told me who did the cut. I got the placenta out and the bleeding controlled and went to work repairing the cut. I had one ER nurse assist me and another listening outside the curtain. I again asked her who cut her, and she again said the people from the People's School. When I called the DA he was delighted because he now had probable cause to get a search warrant and get into the People's School. They were looking for the instrument that was used for the illegal surgery and evidence of the illegal practice of medicine.

The sheriff videotaped the entire search, which revealed examine tables, bloody gloves in the trash, narcotics and dangerous drugs such as Pitocin as well as IV equipment. They also found the group had stolen a Medicaid billing number and were billing the state for deliveries and other things. The tapes were shown to a number of physicians in the local community, and they were asked if they thought this constituted the practice of medicine, which of course they did. My name as the complainant was withheld for fear of harassment.

In the end they were only fined and reached a plea agreement that they would no longer remain in the county and that was it. I was a little disappointed that more wasn't done as we had heard about several small graves about the county as a result of their activities. But as I had previously seen, law enforcement wasn't always vigorous there.

Early on I got to learn that when it comes to malpractice, you can't trust anyone. I had a young couple who had come to me for obstetrical care and seemed pleased with their delivery. I have to admit to some prejudice against circumcision because in those days it was done with one of a couple of clamps, which crushed the foreskin without anesthetic, but this couple wanted it done, so I complied. Shortly thereafter I received notice they wanted to sue me because they didn't think I had cut off enough of the baby's foreskin. The malpractice company got involved, and the next thing I knew, I got a call from a restaurant in the next town that they had a folder of mine. When I got it, I found it was the malpractice company's case file, which had been left in the restaurant by the young woman investigator. Eventually the company gave the couple $1,200 to use to get the child re-circumcised when he grew up if he so desired. After everything was said and done, I found this couple was on my schedule again, and I called them and said after they had sued me, I didn't feel I could be totally objective in their care and suggested they find another doc. Many people don't seem to understand that when they sue a doctor for malpractice, the doctor feels it's extremely personal.

I had never considered myself to be naïve but I must have been. I had a patient who was from Brazil who came in for a vaginal problem. During the visit, she mentioned she was having marital problems because her husband couldn't satisfy her "hot Brazilian blood." Failing to see where this was going, I suggested a marriage or sex counselor. The next time she came in much the same conversation occurred, and I finally was becoming suspicious where this was going. By her third visit nothing was left to chance; as I was sitting on my exam stool writing a prescription, I heard some rustling, and when I looked up, she was reclining on one elbow on the exam table totally nude in a Marilyn Monroe type of pose. I shot out the door and told my assistant to get her dressed and out of the office. I had the receptionist make a note that when this patient called in the future, I was to be totally booked, and she should be shuttled off the female doc I had recently hired. That seemed to result in an immediate cure for her vaginal problems.

Particularly in a small office privacy is always a difficult problem. The way my office was built, the last exam room had a window into a tiny garden, which was surrounded by a privacy fence. One day I came in to do an annual exam on a lady only to find her huddled in a corner next to the window with her paper drape around her. I asked her what the problem was, and she told me there was a man peering over the privacy fence. When I went outside I discovered there had been a roof leak in another office and the roofers were there to repair it. One of the roofers' employees had discovered the windows and was making good use of them. I called the roofer over and explained this was totally unacceptable, and if he couldn't control his employees, I'd call the management company and get him fired. That seemed to solve the problem.

One day I was getting a little bored with routine office work and asked my assistants why it seemed women like those in *Playboy* never seemed to need exams. She just laughed, but the next day there was a new patient in one of the exam rooms whose complaint was that she had some vaginal bleeding after she and her boyfriend had intercourse in an unusual position. When I went into the room, the woman sitting on the exam table with a paper gown on could easily have made Hugh Heffner's top ten. I managed to go ahead with the interview and did the necessary exam, but when I came out of the room, the secretaries and my assistant were in the hall grinning like a gaggle of Cheshire cats. It seemed this lady had come in to make her appointment, and the receptionist had seen her. The receptionist overheard my comment the previous day and had moved the patient's appointment up. They were all waiting for my response, and I assured them I would never complain again.

Things were reaching the point where I was so busy I couldn't keep up. There was a young physician in town who was with the Public Health Service and worked at a clinic sponsored by one of the local Indian tribes. His wife was also a physician, so I talked to her about working for me a couple days a week and she agreed. This allowed me to be open on Saturday but also required the hiring of some additional staff. I also began to look into the possibility of starting a group practice since I had never really wanted to remain in solo practice.

I had originally hoped to have a group office with two of my former junior residents, but when they came to look, we had one of our frequent coastal fogs and the next town on their list was inland in Oregon, which was bright and sunny, and I lost their interest. That didn't change my interest in getting out of solo practice, so I began to explore office possibilities and spent some time looking with a couple of other docs. When we didn't find anything available, it became apparent I'd have to get something built. The hospital owned several acres and the owner was willing to let me have a small plot but only large enough for three docs and no room for expansion. In addition there were restrictions on lab and x-ray to prevent competition so I felt this would not be a long-term solution. I finally found a builder who wanted to build a building and lease it back. He found a piece of land just across the freeway, and on a handshake, he bought it and started building. This meant I had to have the group lined up so we could start immediately when the building was done in order to have enough money to pay the rent. So I began my first venture in recruiting.

My first recruit told me later he and his wife wondered what they'd gotten themselves into when I picked them up at the airport because I was driving my pickup (a stretch cab) and wearing my large black cowboy hat. We got along fine, and he had great credentials having gotten a PhD in psychology and having been in Vietnam as a psychologist before returning to med school and going through a residency in Family Practice. He told me not only were his patients "crazy," but most of his colleagues were as well, so he decided on medicine instead. The only problem was that he needed to work as soon as he got out of residency. We decided we could both work out of my office working four days weekly with the office open six days weekly.

Another recruit was a woman who was just finishing my old residency. She even had the added advantage of a husband who was a lab tech, and since we had a good-sized lab planned in the new building, he was willing to help plan and set that up.

While this woman was there I interviewed another physician who was a pediatrician. They were both at my house for dinner, and after dinner we were sitting and talking when the pediatrician noticed Vinh. He kept trying to get Vinh to stand on his atrophied and paralyzed legs never once realizing he was dealing with a paraplegic. Needless to say he was not hired. The lady was however.

We had room for three docs in addition to me, and our third was an Ob-Gyn who also was finishing a Master of Public Health. He had been in Oakland getting his masters and working doing rape exams for the ER there. He too needed to work immediately when he finished his course, so I was able to arrange for him to rent a small office downtown, which was owned by the hospital, until our building was finished. He advised us he was marrying his girlfriend of two years because he was concerned a small town wouldn't like his current arrangements. A big mistake as we'll see later.

I was approached to be a preceptor for a nurse practice student, and I agreed to take one on. I was credentialed by UC Davis, and my first student was a lady who had always done public health nursing but did have a master's degree. Because she had not had much experience with acute medicine, I tried to get her into the middle of it.

One day an elderly man came in with the strange complaint that he couldn't get his mail. His story was that he had a postal mail box with a combination lock. The box was up high, and every time he went to open it, he would forget the number and sometimes he fainted. I had him show me what he did, and he demonstrated tilting his head up acutely to get his bifocals to focus on the box. I suspected this had something to do with his carotid arteries being put on stretch. We got an urgent ultrasound to see if the artery was being obstructed in extension, but nothing showed up. The next consideration was a Sick Sinus Syndrome. The carotid sinus is located in the carotid artery just behind the angle of the jaw and has a stretch receptor in it. Sometimes this receptor becomes overly sensitive. The purpose of the receptor is to recognize excessive blood pressure, and when stimulated, this slows the heart and lowers the blood pressure. In order to test this we put the man in the hospital, and I got the new young internist on staff to stand by with me. We connected the patient to a heart monitor and then lightly rubbed his carotid sinus. Normally this would slow the heart rate somewhat, but in his case his heart stopped completely. We waited for it to restart, but after thirteen seconds, the internist gave him a thump on the chest, which restarted him. We heard another thump and found my student passed out at the foot of the bed where she'd been watching. We got the chest surgeon to put a pacemaker in the patient, which would take over if his heart stopped, and our patient could once again get his mail.

Insurance companies are one of the necessary evils we had to deal with, and at times they can be totally unreasonable. I had one young man come in complaining that he couldn't buy life insurance to protect his young family because his previous physician had told the company he had diabetes. I got the old records and found that indeed on a single test he was reported to have an elevated blood sugar. No additional testing had been done, and the young man had been diagnosed with diabetes although no treatment was undertaken. I ran several tests including a six-hour tolerance test, several fasting sugars, and found absolutely no evidence of diabetes. The young man also had no symptoms ascribable to diabetes. I put all this in a letter to the insurance company together with my professional opinion that there had been an error in his previous diagnosis. They refused to change their opinion since there is always a question "have you ever been turned down for insurance" on the application forms. He was apparently never going to get insurance from anyone in spite of filing an appeal with my support.

The state of California, like most states, has a panel of physicians who evaluate disability claims. They sent me a letter asking if I would do some evaluations for them, and I felt I should do my share. The ground rules were that I could only evaluate but not treat. The first patient I saw came in in a wheelchair with a long list of very serious problems he thought he had, including MS and diabetes. I started methodically to evaluate each disorder, and as each came up negative, he would drop whatever behavior went with that complaint. By the time we'd completed the evaluation with *no* illness found, he'd started at the local junior college and no longer used his wheelchair.

The next patient to be evaluated was a woman who seemed severely depressed. I told the state she was indeed disabled by her severe depression, but if properly treated probably would be able to return to work. I was myself depressed knowing she would probably go on like that when she could easily be treated if she had the right physician.

One day I heard a commotion in the waiting room and went to see what was happening. I found the son of a local politician with a dart game dart stuck in the bridge of his nose. I took him back and removed the dart, cleaned the wound, and put him on antibiotics. He never had any problems from it but certainly shocked my waiting room.

Another new patient came in refusing to tell my assistant what he wanted. When I got in the room, it turned out he had a flashlight stuck in his rectum. When I did his exam I was able to hook a corner of the tube with my gloved finger and remove it. We went ahead and did a proctoscope to ensure there was no perforation. He never to my knowledge came back, probably something to do with embarrassment. This isn't all that rare. The chief instruments were vibrators, flashlights, and carrots. Our surgeon had a corkscrew welded on a stainless rod to use to remove carrots after we had to remove one in little pieces when we couldn't grasp it through the colonoscope. I saw one surgeon remove a light bulb using forceps designed for premature infants. He managed to do this without breaking the bulb.

A few weeks later the daughter of the same politician whose son had the dart in his nose was brought in by the mother with an overdose. She was thirteen and very dramatic. She'd gotten into a fight with her parents and had proceeded to take an entire bottle of Tylenol (100). Since this drug is a liver poison, it doesn't do anything immediately obvious, so she just went to bed, but when she woke she began vomiting and finally told her mother what she had done. I admitted her to the ICU and called poison control. Her blood levels were in the fatal range and she was past the twelve hours in which they knew the antidote worked, but we decided there was nothing to lose by trying. The antidote was always in the hospital because it was also used in breathing treatments to loosen mucus so we gave her the recommended dose. I had to tell her parents that she might well die from this and we could only wait. As time progressed, she seemed to stabilize and her liver enzymes quit rising. Within a day or two it was apparent she was getting rapidly better and I was able to discharge her with a recommendation that she get psychological help.

Poison control called daily at first to see what happened, and now the recommendation is to use the antidote if the ingestion is within twenty-four hours.

OB took off when we opened our doors, and we quickly realized it would have to be limited if I were going to survive. I decided I could handle about ten deliveries a month, and while tiring this seemed to be possible. The one month my schedulers lost track, I ended up with almost twenty deliveries scheduled. That was a very rough month.

The group practice building was finally in the finishing stages and we started to get everyone moved in. The obstetrician brought his receptionist and we had to hire several assistants.

Group Practice

As our new building neared completion, the OB and I went to see how things were coming along. They had told us the alarm wasn't connected to the telephone yet, but they had temporarily hooked it to a siren so we decided to test it. I put the key in the alarm and we opened the door. The OB walked into the building, and about ten feet in, the siren went off. It was inside and was so loud it put him on his knees. I was laughing so hard it was hard to turn it off. The building was progressing nicely except all the exam room doors were mounted backward. Doors on exam rooms are supposed to open toward the side wall, which is just the reverse from all others, but it keeps people in the hall from seeing into the room as you go in and out. The contractor corrected the problem and shortly thereafter we moved in.

We had staff for most positions but needed to hire additional people because our woman doctor had been working ERs while waiting on the building and had no assistant. One young lady applied and had very good credentials but had been out of work for some months because of a neck injury. I was concerned about this problem, but we hired her and she turned out to be one of the most faithful employees we ever had. It turned out she competed in rodeos on the weekends and would get injured occasionally but never missed work because of it. She would bring her horse to work on Fridays and tether it beside her horse trailer for the day where it would munch the grass at the edge of our employee parking area. As soon as work was ended, she'd take off to whichever rodeo she had scheduled. Eventually she married a cowboy and moved to Wyoming, which, I think, was what she'd always wanted.

Our receptionist had been the hospital telephone operator and was a local resident, so she knew nearly everybody in town and would call them by their names as they came in. One day I heard her screaming at a man for bleeding on our new rugs, so I went to see what was going on. I found an old farmer with his pants leg torn from his knee to his groin and his leg open from just above the knee to inches from his scrotum. We got temporary dressings on him to control the bleeding and took him to the hospital. I had to explain to him this was more serious than a few stitches in the office. His story was that he and his dog were moving a boar to a sow's pen for breeding when the boar decided not to cooperate. He'd gotten the old man in the leg with a tusk and ripped him to the bone but fortunately missed the great vessels in the leg. I asked where the boar was now, fearing additional injuries, but he said he'd gone home and got a gun and "shot the SOB" before he came in. I took him to the OR where I closed the muscles with drains in place, anticipating infection from what I told him was probably not a sterile tusk. After three days of sterile wet dressings, I closed the skin with a drain in place and let him go from the hospital. He eventually healed just fine. I suspect he learned to move the sow to the boar after that unless he had more help.

When a patient came to the ER who didn't have a physician, the backup physician was expected to do follow-up or admission if needed. Backup was rotated among all the physicians in a particular specialty. One day I was on backup when a young hippy-looking girl came in with a knee that was red and swollen and so sore she could barely bear weight. She was going to have to be admitted for her septic (infected) joint and had no physician. On admission I found only a heavy yellow vaginal discharge, which was suspicious for gonorrhea. The lab confirmed my suspicion, and when I needled her knee, I got thick pus, which also had organisms that looked like gonococcus (GC). I flushed the joint and instilled an antibiotic and got her admitted. I asked our orthopedic surgeon to take a look, and he recommended daily tapping and intra joint antibiotics in addition to the IV antibiotics I was also giving her. The infection was very slow to respond, and I had finally placed a tube in the joint and would flush it out with antibiotic solution. After ten days we were still getting about 50 cc of pus daily from the joint when Medicaid advised us she had to be discharged. I called the physician at the Medi-Cal (California

Medicaid) office and explained that while she was doing better, I felt if we stopped her treatment, the infection would come right back. He was adamant that the book said ten days and that was all we could get. I asked for his name and he wanted to know why. I told him I wanted to give it to the patient, so when she lost her knee joint, she would know whom to sue. At that point he decided maybe we could have more time after all, but he insisted I get an orthopedic consult. I told him that since the orthopedic surgeon had been looking in on her case the entire time, I was delighted he would get paid for his time. She continued to get better and eventually was discharged but not until after making a pass at me, which I really found to be obnoxious.

I had one older lady come in who said she hadn't been able to get along with her doctors in the past. She really was hard to deal with, but she also exhibited the symptoms of depression, and I was able to convince her to try an antidepressant. When I saw her again in a couple weeks, she was remarkably different and very much improved. She became a long-time patient, but we had to supply her meds from the sample closet because she had very little money and no insurance.

One day I got a call from the ER that this lady's husband had been brought in by ambulance after he'd rolled a truck on a freeway exit. When I got there, I found he was in pretty good shape except his head had gone through the open side window, and the roadway had scalped him. Fortunately the scalp was still there but had been peeled back from about the hairline in the front to the apex of the scull and up to the midline. He really wasn't bleeding as badly as I expected, so I took him to the OR and cleaned his wound with lots of flushing. I found he had gravel embedded in the skull and the only way I could remove it was with a bone rasp (similar to a file but with much larger teeth). Once he was cleaned up, I placed drains in the open areas and closed the scalp. We applied a pressure dressing to keep fluid from accumulating and admitted him for IV antibiotics. He did very well and I was able to remove the drains and send him home in a few days. He proceeded to heal without incident, and since the lacerations had been in the hair line, they weren't even visible.

Our office became so busy it was getting hard to keep up. One day I was assisting our Ob-Gyn with a couple of scheduled hysterectomies when I was called that a patient of mine had come in in labor. He had a scheduled C-section to do, so we found someone else from the office to assist him while I went to check on my patient. When I examined her, I found she was dilating with the head still floating, and I could feel the cord in front of the head. This can lead to a disaster if the head traps the cord as it comes down, cutting off the oxygen to the baby. She needed an immediate C-section. In those days we had to use the OR; whereas, today most facilities can do a C-section in the delivery room. As we moved her down, I found a GP friend of mine in the hallway and asked him to assist me. The surgery went without a hitch and mom and baby were back to OB for postpartum care. By the time we added them up, we had done seven or eight major surgeries that day including an ectopic pregnancy after the C-sections. We were just finishing getting our orders written at about 11:00 p.m. when the ER called with another vaginal bleeder. Ultrasound and pregnancy test ruled out ectopic pregnancy, but she was bleeding fast enough he thought she needed a D and C. We both were so tired, we didn't feel safe so we started her on IV estrogen, which slowed the bleeding and went home to sleep. When we stopped the estrogen the next day, she began hemorrhaging again and he did her D and C, which got it under control.

One young woman came in with her two-year-old to get a burn dressing changed, which had been applied in the ER the night before. I looked at the burn pattern and asked the mother how this had happened. She said her boyfriend had been babysitting while she worked the evening shift as a waitress, and the baby had reached for a cup of coffee on the table. I had to tell her the pattern of the burn didn't match the story, and by California law I had to report my suspicion of child abuse. When the police arrived, I told them of my suspicions, and they went in to talk to the mother. They ran out and left my parking lot with their lights and sirens going. When I talked to them later, they told me they knew the boyfriend and he had just gotten out of prison for flinging a baby into a wall and killing it. When I later talked with the DA, I explained why the burn pattern was not from an accidental burn. The burn pattern involved all four fingers *and the thumb* in a circumferential burn. If the child had reached for the cup, the thumb wouldn't be involved. In addition if the child's hand hadn't been controlled, it would have been suddenly withdrawn and this was usually associated "splash" burns when the cup was overturned. There were no splash burns.

The DA told me they were filing misdemeanor child abuse against the boyfriend. I was totally confused, but he said the prior record couldn't be presented in court, and the only testimony would be mine. Apparently they were too cheap to hire another expert to look at the evidence. They felt that he would plead to the misdemeanor, and at least they would get a second conviction on his record. I didn't see what good that would do since it was only admissible for sentencing, but that was the way things went down. I testified at the arraignment and the judge bound him over for trial; then he copped a plea. At least he wasn't going to be babysitting that child any more. It was hard to believe the mother was that naïve in the first place.

We were constantly on the alert for child abuse and the law was very specific that if we failed to report even a suspicion of child abuse, we could be held liable. On the other hand, we could not be sued if it turned out we were wrong. One mother brought in a four-year-old for a burn. When I examined the child, I found multiple burns of varying ages and at varying stages of healing. This is supposed to be one of the major red flags in a pediatric exam. We dressed the burn, and then I told the mother we would have to have her home checked to see if someone was burning her child. She said they were living in a very small house and the only heat was a wood stove in the middle of the living room and the child would run into the stove every so often. I called Child Protective Services, and the worker took a sheriff with her. When I saw her later I ask what she had found and she started laughing. She said they had a tiny house with the stove in the middle of the living room just as described, and indeed the CPS worker had brushed against the stove and burned herself.

Although we were very busy, we were also able to have some lighter moments. One day the back office assistants made up a fake chart for the last patient, which they put it up for our woman physician. The patients name was I. M. Studly, and the complaint was listed as impotence. When she opened the chart to look at past history there was a Playgirl centerfold pasted in.

Most of the office didn't know our FP/Psychologist had written his PhD thesis on the use of humor in therapy. One day the typist came out of her booth laughing and handed around the dictation she had just finished typing about a man who came in wearing a skin-tight suit with a big "S" in his chest. He claimed to be faster than a speeding bullet and able to leap tall buildings in a single bound. The final diagnosis was megalomania. Not long thereafter, another dictation came in about a girl who claimed to be a princess and allegedly lived with seven dwarves. The final diagnosis on that was nymphomania.

The hardest part of the group practice was managing it, and this required frequent meetings of the physicians who were owners. One time the OB invited us to meet at his house, which was a beautiful Victorian mansion in town. He had been fortunate enough to get to rent this landmark. We had known he and his new wife weren't getting along as well as one would hope, but we had no idea how bad things were until we were sitting there talking when she came storming in and kicked his dog, which was lying there. He immediately jumped up and ran after her, and we were afraid we were going to witness a murder right there. Fortunately they just engaged in a shouting match in the next room, and we cancelled the rest of the meeting and never held one at his house again.

By this time I had another nurse practice student who had been a neonatal ICU nurse but wanted to do outpatient-medicine. She asked me to look at a patient she'd just seen with flu-like symptoms. This young woman was from New Guinea and was just visiting friends in our area before returning home. She had been at the University of Nebraska and had just finished up. My student thought she looked too sick to have a run-of-the-mill virus. Since she was a visitor and looked so ill, we decided to admit her to the hospital. The admission physical showed what appeared to be an enlarged heart. The x-ray showed a "water bottle heart," which is a shape associated with pericardial fluid (fluid in the space between the heart and its surrounding membrane). The ultrasound confirmed the presence of fluid in this space. This can be very dangerous since as pressure builds up, the heart can no longer fill properly, and the patient can suffer sudden death. I consulted with the chest surgeon, and we did a pericardial tap to remove the fluid and sent it for culture and cellular exam and left a tube in place to prevent further buildup. I sent out cultures of sputum, blood, and urine and sent viral cultures to the state as well. We put the patient in the ICU for observation. The next day we found the pericardial tube had gotten pulled out, and fluid appeared to be re-accumulating, so the chest surgeon was reluctant to try to put another tube in place. We took her to the OR where he stripped the pericardium so fluid couldn't accumulate and cultured the pericardium and nearby lung as well as getting pathology of those tissues. Post op I got a call from the ICU that the patient had spiked a fever to 108°F, which was confirmed by electronic thermometer and the nurses had packed the patient in ice. We also started her on acetaminophen since aspirin is an anticoagulant and is not a good idea immediately post op. I was hoping this was just a post-anesthetic fever when she spiked again and got to 106°F before the nurses got it under control. Our local infectious disease specialist had nothing to add, so at that point I called the chief of infectious disease at Stanford and told him about the case. He agreed to accept the patient there and see if they could figure it out. After the transfer I would get daily calls from the resident on the case to check on our cultures. He told me they were stumped, and the infectious disease people thought maybe it was an inflammatory disease like Lupus, but the inflammatory disease specialists said it wasn't and were convinced it was infectious. She slowly got better and they sent her back without a diagnosis. We held her a few days, but since she seemed completely recovered, we allowed her to continue her journey. She apparently was fine because we got a Christmas card from her the next year.

One patient had started with me in solo practice working on her weight. When we started, she weighed about 525 pounds. With hypnotherapy we eventually got her down to about 400 pounds but seemed unable to progress beyond that. I saw her for all the other problems her extreme obesity caused, such as diabetes, but she had been stable for several years when she called the office and told one of my partners she just wasn't feeling well. He worked her in just after lunch, but when she should have been coming in, her husband called to say he'd come home for lunch and found her dead. We later saw research on extreme obesity that told of similar deaths in the hospital, which appeared to be cardiac in origin. As far as I know little is understood about this even today.

I seemed to be off duty when my patients called for urgent slots. One of my patients called complaining of bad heart burn and was brought in to see my partner since I was off that day. My last note in the timber company executive's chart was that I had warned him if he didn't stop smoking and start taking his blood pressure meds, he was due to have a heart attack. Indeed he just sat down in the waiting room when he keeled over onto the rug. He had had a cardiac arrest. We had a "crash cart" for just such an emergency, and while my partners worked on the patient, our nurses brought the cart. The cart had been made up of one of those rolling tool chests Sear's sells and had an interlock, which wouldn't allow the drawers to open if the top was down. In the excitement my partner forgot about the interlock but was so full of adrenaline he opened the drawer anyway. When I came in later there were little pieces of metal on the rug in the waiting room from the drawer lock. Unfortunately my patient expired and they couldn't get him back.

I had one lady who, while in labor, had severe depressions (slowing) in fetal heart rate, and we rushed her to the OR for a C-section. When we got the baby out, it had a "scaphoid abdomen," which means it is sucked inward rather than being the usual protuberant tummy associated with babies. My colleague who was acting as pediatrician also was having trouble breathing for it. This combination usually means the child's diaphragm hasn't formed right, and the gut is in the chest. The x-ray confirmed this diagnosis and we called the surgeon to see if we could improve the situation. He felt we needed to immediately get the gut back where it belonged and began setting up for surgery in the next OR. I finished closing the Cesarean and had my assistant finish the skin while I went into the adjacent OR to help the surgeon. We found the leaflets of the left diaphragm had not fused and were on the side wall of the chest under a small membrane. We got all the bowel back in the abdomen and redeveloped the leaflets and took down a small membrane, which was on the collapsed lung and closed the diaphragm. We were able to get the abdomen closed although it was tight. Often it is necessary to put in a piece of Dacron to close the abdomen because it hasn't stretched enough to hold all the abdominal contents. I contacted the neonatologist at Oakland Children's Hospital and told him what we had. Up to this point we were barely able to move enough air and maintain the pH of the blood at barely acceptable levels. The infant was transported by aircraft to Oakland and did OK for two or three days when it suddenly went downhill and died. The mother was devastated, but she was young and fertile and would be able to try again although that didn't alleviate her grief at the time.

One night I was in the hospital finishing a delivery about 4:00 a.m. when the ER called to say the ER physician would like me to come down because they had a severe injury coming in in mild shock. When I got there, the ambulance was just driving in, and they were carrying a man I knew to be the boyfriend of one of our office assistants. He worked nightshift at one of the local paper mills. His job was to run the chipper, which took logs and chipped them up to use to make pulp. Apparently the machine had jammed and he had turned it off but had forgotten and left the key in. While he had his arm in the chipper to clear the jam, some idiot had turned it on. His arm was removed just below the elbow and he had lost quite a bit of blood. While we got the bleeding under control, I sent the ambulance back to the mill to fetch the arm and hand. We had those cooled just short of frostbite, and then I called the transplant team in San Francisco and advised them what we had. By this time the patient was stable, so we sent patient and arm down by air ambulance. They called me later in the morning to say the tendons had been pulled out rather than cleanly cut and they couldn't put the arm back on so they just completed the closing of the amputation and sent him back. He later opted for a hook prosthesis and became the best at operating that device I'd ever seen. He also married my medical assistant and she quit to be a housewife. I forgave him, however, and we were friends for many years thereafter.

I was called in the middle of the night about the father of one of my patients who was visiting and had developed severe chest pain. When I went in I found an elderly man writhing with pain, which he described as a tearing quality. His ECG had been done by the ER staff before I arrived and did not show an injury pattern. His chest x-ray did show thickening of the aortic root, and on physical exam he had very pale eye grounds (instead of the usual red color) in the right eye. I asked the internist on call to take a look as well and he agreed with my findings, indicating the man had a dissecting aortic aneurysm starting at the root of the aorta. These are usually the result of arteriosclerosis with the inner part of the vessel wall separating from the outer part.

This is made worse by high blood pressure, and we started the man on medications to lower his blood pressure as low as was safe. Our chest surgeon had trained in UC Davis, and we asked him to look. Since we didn't have the heart-lung machine necessary to deal with this problem during surgery, he called his old mentor who agreed to take the patient in transfer and have his team standing by. We sent him down with a nurse to manage the blood pressure med, and he arrived fine, but when his arteriogram was done there, the dissection had re-canalized (opened back into the main channel at the end) and it was thought the surgery was more dangerous than just leaving things as they were. His daughter told me a couple years later he was continuing to do well with carefully controlled blood pressure.

One young lady came for OB care, and I found that she had a vaginal septum, which consisted of a string of normal tissue extending from the top of the vagina to the posterior forchette (midline). This went easily to the side and was not full length up to the cervix so I thought it would not be a big problem. Her pregnancy went normally until about the twenty-sixth week when she came in in hard labor. We were unable to get the contractions to stop so when the head came down I took her to the delivery room where I found the head had the vaginal septum holding it up. I couldn't work the head to one side or the other, so I just put clamps on the string of tissue and divided it to allow the child to deliver. The baby was very small weighing in at exactly one kilogram (2.2 pounds) including an umbilical catheter and a breathing tube. I tied off the septal pieces and got the placenta delivered rapidly and turned my attention to the infant. Her color was good, and when I got the umbilical catheter placed her pH and oxygen were good as well. I placed a nasotracheal tube as a precaution in case she started to develop fetal lung syndrome. I then called UC San Francisco to request transfer only to be told by the neonatal fellow that they had no neonatal beds and as far as he knew that was the case for the whole city. The only suggestion he had was that one of their attending neonatologists had a three-bed NICU and I could call him. When I talked to him and told him the story, he was amazed and asked if I was boarded in both Ob-Gyn and Pediatrics, and I had to tell him I was just a country FP. I had called the pediatricians in the next town, but they had refused to come, saying the infant was too premature to survive anyway. When Marin County Hospital agreed to accept the transfer, I had my nurse practice student come in to care for the baby while I got things arranged (remember this lady was an experienced NICU nurse). Usually when we transferred a sick infant, the university would send up a plane equipped with an incubator as well as a NICU nurse and a neonatal fellow, but Marin didn't have such amenities. The only neonatal transport incubator was at one of the hospitals in the next town, and when I called to ask to borrow it, they refused because they didn't know when they might need it. I contacted our hospital administrator who called their administrator and advised him that we would sue if the baby died before we could arrange transfer. They decided we could borrow the unit, and I sent my nurse along to monitor the baby as needed. She told me later the ambulance that was supposed to meet her plane didn't show up, and she ended up on the tarmac with a tiny baby in an incubator. They finally showed up and the rest of the transfer went smoothly. The neonatologist called me daily to report progress, which was great. The baby never had any problems. After a week or so, the baby was transferred back to us as she only needed tube feeding until she got big enough to suckle, and we could handle that. This also allowed her mother to be with her and help with her care.

At the postpartum visit I told the mother she probably had a septum in her uterus as well, and we needed to get a hysterogram to determine if this could be repaired. She didn't get the workup but rather showed up pregnant soon after. I explained to her if things got crowded because of a septum in the uterus she could go into premature labor again and she needed to rest when she got over twenty weeks. Instead, when she was again about twenty-six weeks, I got a call from a physician in Oregon wanting to confirm her story and saying she was there camping when she went into labor. Later I heard she delivered in a helicopter on her way to a medical center up there, and the baby died. She never came back to me again, which was just as well as I wasn't feeling very sympathetic. Over the years I did see the baby I delivered around town apparently doing well.

I got a call one day to come see a patient in OB who was at term and bleeding more heavily than usual. When I got there the patient turned out to be the very obese daughter of one of our ER nurses. The girl was about five feet tall and weighed about 230 pounds. An emergency ultrasound showed the placenta over the opening of the cervix. This is called a placenta previa and can be fatal for both mother and child, so I immediately took her to the OR where we were able to deliver a healthy baby by C-section. The post-op period was uneventful, but I did stress to her that if she was thinking about getting pregnant in the future, she needed to lose weight. She never seemed to take that advice very seriously.

One night our lady physician called me to see if I could help her with a difficult delivery. The baby was in the occiput posterior position. Normally babies deliver with the face toward the mother's back but once in a while they get turned the wrong direction and this makes delivery very difficult because the narrowest diameter of the head can't approach the birth canal. I came in and was able to turn the baby with my fingers, which were much stronger than hers. The delivery went ahead normally, and after everything was done, we were free to go home. When the hospital was built, there were only male physicians so there was only one dressing room to change out of your greens (scrub suit). We walked into the dressing room discussing the case and were both in our underwear before we realized what was happening. I figured she was just another physician, and I guess she must have come to the same conclusion so we both continued to get dressed and nothing was ever said.

Our area was the place the hippie movement went when Haight-Ashbury became a tourist area. We had a central square in town where some of the less desirable characters hung out at night, and this fellow was one of them. He'd been drinking wine with his friends when they got into an argument, and one of them stuck him with an ice pick. I was called to help the surgeon. Externally the wound wasn't impressive, but he obviously had something wrong internally. When we opened the abdomen, we found his stomach distended with wine, and if there was any pressure on it, wine would squirt out like it was coming from a Bota Bag. We decided he didn't need to absorb more wine, and it was making it more difficult to repair. The anesthesiologist passed a naso-gastric tube and drained about a quart of wine from his stomach. We were then able to over-sew the hole. Nothing else was punctured so we went ahead and closed. The patient did well post op.

Because of the hippie population, marijuana was the major crop in the area and was used fairly openly. There was a theater downtown where they allowed smoking and the smell was rarely tobacco. My wife and I went to a movie there and both felt a little light-headed by the end. One young woman was in the office for a routine annual exam, and when I read her history form, she listed her occupation as farmer. Since we had a number of organic farms in the area, I asked her what she grew; she replied marijuana. I guess my poker face slipped because she explained that she knew I wasn't going to turn her in, and she was tired of lying about it. She told me it was her third year, and if she got away with it one more time, she would retire and do her art the rest of her life (she was an art student) and never have to worry about money. She said she was clearing over $100,000 a year and, of course, not paying taxes.

We had a new young surgeon come in, and he told me shortly after he started he was on ER backup when he was called for a young man on Medi-Cal (who was probably a marijuana grower) with an appendicitis. He said he removed the appendix, and when the man came into the office to get his stitches out, he asked about the bill. The young surgeon said he would just wait until Medi-Cal sent payment, but the young man insisted he wanted to pay so the surgeon told him the charge was $650. The young man pulled out a roll of $100 bills and counted off seven of them. The surgeon explained he was just starting out in practice and didn't have that much change on hand. The young man told him to keep the change and left. The surgeon told me nobody had told him in residency about surgeons being tipped.

Another of our young hippies gave me a scare. We had been seeing HIV for some years, and it was just beginning to show up in our female population. This was largely from drug use and needle sharing. I was called to the ER as backup to sew up a wound in a patient's hand, which the ER doctor didn't have time to do. The young woman was barefoot with multiple rings on her toes and wearing a nearly floor-length hand-woven skirt and tie-dye shirt. Her laceration was in her fourth finger and clearly needed stitches. I normally put in a nerve block for digits and had started to put one in her finger when she slapped at my hand driving the needle through her finger and into my other hand, which was holding hers so I could judge the depth of the needle. I had never had an adult do anything like that before, and my first thought was that if there ever was a woman who might be using injectible drugs or sleeping with a drug user, this was her. Fortunately all her tests were negative, but I was really a nervous wreck until the results came back. I did complete her repair after getting her numb. The second time she held absolutely rigid.

Sue had still wanted to have her own pregnancy and had been going to an infertility specialist in the next town. I knew his history and knew he'd come from being a chief at an eastern medical school. He'd had a drinking problem and was fired. Two Ob-Gyns in the next town had recruited him, but rumor said he'd gone back to drinking. With his help Sue got pregnant and decided she would go to him for prenatal care. When she finally came to term, she went into the hospital in the next town where she had a very desultory labor. One of his partners came and ruptured her membrane, which puts a deadline since you would normally want to deliver the infant within twenty-four hours to avoid infection. When her doctor came in to check her in the evening, she wasn't making much progress. He mentioned it was his anniversary, and I could smell alcohol on his breath already. It was about 10:00 p.m. and he was going home. I told him I didn't want him drinking in case something happened and suggested he sleep in the physician's lounge down the hall because if he tried to leave and go drinking there would be physical consequences. He apparently realized I meant it and stayed the night. In the morning she still was not close to delivery, so they went to C-Section while I went for a walk. Mother and new daughter were fine and I finally went home after being up a total of fifty-one hours, which was my record.

This man was involved with our group once more. His partners apparently had called him in and told him he either had to go to rehab and stop drinking or they were going to have to fire him. They even offered to pay for the rehab. He went to the hospital and did a scheduled exploratory laparoscope and then drove to the beach and blew his head off with a shotgun. He hadn't dictated his op note so no one knew what he'd seen in the scope. The patient was our Ob's wife.

I had one lady whose baby had a disproportionately large head, but we could see no hydrocephalus (excess fluid in the brain). When she went into labor, the head wouldn't even descend into the pelvis so we had to go to C-section. When I delivered the infant from the uterus, it was obvious what was going on. The baby had all the findings of the most common kind of dwarfism (achondroplastic dwarf). The baby would probably have normal intelligence but would be small with a disproportionately large head and short limbs. She seemed to tolerate it well, and I suggested she contact Little People of America, which helps such families. The child grew as expected and did well.

Having a large practice with several docs doing OB can result in some confusion. We tried to have at least one appointment with the other docs who might be doing a patient's delivery so he or she wouldn't be a complete stranger. I got a call at home one night about a patient of one of my partners who was in hard labor. I raced for the hospital and found the nurses had moved her into the delivery room already so I changed and scrubbed rapidly. I asked the nurse what the woman's due date was and she said the fifteenth. Since it was about the tenth of the month, I assumed she was near term (forty weeks). I went into the delivery room and the head was presenting at the vaginal opening. I put my hand across the perineum (tissue between the vagina and the rectum) to support it to prevent tearing when the lady gave a big grunt and this very small baby shot through my fingers, out to the end of the cord, and swung almost to the floor. I grabbed the infant up and dealt with the cord. The room had gone deathly silent, but the baby began a good, lusty cry. The father was there as was the lady's mother. I checked the baby thoroughly and again questioned the nurse about the due date and learned it was the fifteenth of the next month, and the baby was about four or five weeks premature. Mother and child did fine, and the father, instead of being mad, thought it was the funniest thing he had ever seen and nicknamed the baby Rocket in honor of her entrance into the world. When I told one of the older docs about this embarrassment, he just said, "If you haven't dropped one, you haven't done much OB."

I was called to help with a breech presentation, which was unexpected. We occasionally would do a breech delivery, but it was felt to be safer to do a C-section. Since we didn't have much time, we rushed to the OR, but I was fortunate enough to have thought to have the OB nurses bring a set of Piper forceps, which are used in breech deliveries to deliver the after-coming head. As we transferred the woman to the operating table, the breech popped out and there was nothing to do but deliver the baby. I was able to "break down" the breech, which means sweeping a finger to bring the legs out since they are normally up toward the chest. I brought the baby down and asked for the Pipers. The normal application of these is to swing them from below the mom's pelvis and slip them into place, but somehow I was able to apply them on the OR table with the nurses holding the patient's legs and the infant delivered successfully. Mom and baby were fine, but the doctor was a nervous wreck.

I assisted our orthopedic surgeon quite a bit and generally knew what he was going to do on each procedure. I would often be called on New Year's Eve at about 11:00 p.m. to assist with the accident victims that needed surgery. We'd work on getting the fractures set and the rods and plates in place, and then while he did the casting, I would go ahead and sew the facial lacerations, which he avoided. This would often go on all night. Over the years, the state lowered the blood alcohol limit to 0.08 percent and increased the penalties, as well as enforcing seatbelt laws, which decreased our trauma nights quite a bit. I admit it somewhat dampened my own New Year's Eve because I enjoyed the trauma surgery, but it probably did save a lot of lives.

When the orthopedic surgeon was attending medical education meetings or just vacationing, he would hire a senior resident from his old program to cover for him. I guess he'd told the young men they could call me for assistance, and one evening I got such a call to come and assist with a terrible hand injury. The patient was a young woman who had rolled her car on a freeway ramp and had had her arm on the window ledge and her hand gripping the outside of the top of the door. When the car rolled it caught her fingers between the ground and the top of the window crushing them. When I got a look at the wound, I really felt that they were going to have to be amputated. We went to surgery and cleaned the wounds and began to see if there was anything we could save. We both were aware that her history included the fact that she played the violin. As we just went from one problem to the next, the fingers slowly came back together with several tiny wires and pins, and we actually got them repaired. I was extremely impressed with this young resident for saving her fingers and at least giving her a chance to be able to use them again. From there on it depended on PT and rehab and how hard she was willing to work. The fingers healed and the blood supply seemed adequate, but I never heard any long-term follow-up.

Our new young surgeon had a patient who had been admitted to him who was a chronic alcoholic. This man was admitted for gastrointestinal bleeding. These patients bleed from verraces of the esophageal veins (similar to varicose veins in the leg) caused by increased pressure in the enteric circulation. This circulation takes blood from the stomach and intestines to the liver for processing before it gets into the general circulation. The only connections to the general circulation are at the esophagus and the hemorrhoids and when the pressure goes up in this system because of sclerosis (essentially scarring) of the liver the veins on the esophagus and the hemorrhoid veins expand. The result is when these veins in the esophagus start to bleed, the patient can bleed out very quickly. The treatment, if you can't stop the bleeding, is to make a shunt from the enteric system to the general venous system thereby lowering the enteric pressure. I was called because the patient had started to bleed after being stopped and was probably going to continue. He'd had several units of blood but was losing ground. When we got into the abdomen, it turned out he had several anomalous veins, and after dissecting a number of inadequate vessels, we found the only by-pass that would work was to connect the splenic vein to the right renal. This involved placing a Dacron graft, which was a bit of a stretch. We were plodding along when about 4:00 a.m. the young surgeon was ready to quit with the job half done. Anesthesia and I had to coach him through each stitch one at a time until the connection was made and was free of leaks. We finally got through the surgery and post op the patient did well. The surgeon told me later he'd told the patient one more drink could finish him off. He got a thank-you card a few months later from the patient who wasn't drinking probably because he was in the state penitentiary in Montana.

One of my patients brought her sister in to be seen. The lady was a traveling sales person and had developed extreme tiredness. She'd been found to be anemic elsewhere and had seen a rather famous hematologist who simply hadn't been able to figure it out. When I looked at her lab, she did have a severe anemia of the iron-deficiency type. There are two reasons for this state. Either you are not getting enough iron in your diet (or not absorbing it) or you are bleeding somewhere. After her initial physical, I felt sure it was the latter because I could feel a mass in her right abdomen. Tests confirmed there was blood in her stool, and x-rays showed a large mass in her cecum (where the large bowel connects to the small intestine). We took her to surgery and removed the mass, which was, of course, a cancer of the colon. She did well post op, but with a bowel cancer that size penetrating the outer layers of the bowel, we knew that it was just a matter of time. We were very clear with her that we couldn't cure this, and chemotherapy at that time had very little effect on that tumor. She accepted that and showed one of the best attitudes I'd ever seen from a patient with a terminal illness. The next thing I knew she was involved in a course on death and dying at the local JC. Apparently she would shock the class by introducing herself and saying, "I am dying of colon cancer." She was able to keep that up for over two years until a metastasis started to constrict her esophagus, and we had to put a feeding tube down to maintain nutrition. She was starting to have to use more and more morphine to control the pain until one day her sister called for a refill on her morphine and asked for a larger quantity. I was a little suspicious but felt if she'd made her decision, I wasn't about to argue so we filled it. The next day the sister called to tell us she'd died in her sleep.

You think you know your patients pretty well, but sometimes they don't want you to know everything. I had one lady in her early sixties who was brought to the ER with all the symptoms of a stroke. In those days we couldn't do much about the active stroke, so she was admitted and watched before starting physical therapy. She showed signs of recovery but it seemed slow. Her son from a previous marriage had flown in and I was explaining to him that she was doing well but a number of findings seemed to indicate she seemed older than she was. He told me she really was much older than she admitted. She'd subtracted twenty years from her age when she married her current husband and had lied about her age to everyone since. This meant she really was about eighty rather than sixty. We agreed not to tell her husband, and I don't think he ever figured it out. Currently stroke is considered an emergency and should be treated at an ER, which is designated as a stroke center because there is so much that can be done to reverse the problem.

I got to be friends with a Forest Service technician when I delivered his wife. We began to go cutting firewood together. This worked out very well because among his various jobs he was assigned the job of marking the trees deemed to be surplus and available to cut. One time we had cut a tree, and it hung up in the tree next to it, so he went to his truck and got a paint bucket and splashed a line of paint on the tree holding ours up. He said, "I declare this tree surplus" so we cut it down as well. That resulted in a huge load of green fire wood and coming back to the Forest Service road, I hit a small gully and the back of the truck bottomed out. When we got back to the highway, the Forest Service road was coming down a steep incline, and I found the truck didn't want to stop with all that weight. I had to jam on the brakes and skidded to a halt just feet short of the highway, which had loaded logging trucks racing past. I got out to check my load and noticed the spare tire, which hung under the truck, wasn't there. I ended up turning around and going back to the gully where I found my tire. There was a tire-shaped dent in the bottom of my gas tank and the tank lost two gallons of capacity. Afterward all four tires went *thump, thump* down the road until I replaced them with new ones that didn't have flat spots.

Many of our patients didn't have health insurance and didn't qualify for Medi-Cal. Medical care was a major concern for them, and we tried to help where we could. One patient asked if I could use firewood, and since I'd given up on fixing up the house we'd bought originally and since we'd bought a new house which had a fireplace and a wood stove, I was delighted to get a source of firewood. I had been going to the National Forest and cutting my own, but it was a lot of work. This man's wife became a regular patient and was quite a character. She wore a gold pendant of which she was very proud that consisted of a word in cursive writing, which said, "Bitch." After a year or so of this barter arrangement, he came in with a typical chainsaw laceration, which I would see every so often where the men would finish cutting a tree and would rest their heavy saws on their left thighs. Sometimes they did this without waiting for the blade to quit running. The result was an oblique laceration of the anterior thigh down to or into the muscle. Since a chain takes a large kerf (the width of the cut), these were usually messy. I fixed his leg and got six cords of wood. The only stipulation was that I had to go to his cabin in the mountains and pick it up because he couldn't afford the gas.

When I drove up in the mountains to get some of my wood, the patient showed me a huge stack of wood, which was mine, and he said I could come get it any time whether they were there or not. They lived in a log cabin made from the local wood, and the woman was very proud they had just installed running water although the restroom was still out back. This guy was a real mountain man who trapped in the winter and cut firewood and worked on his place in the summer. They had about eighty acres and were almost self-sufficient. The ceiling of his cabin had guns hanging from it, many of them antiques he inherited from his grandfather.

I had one man who paid his bills in fence posts (we built a lovely three-rail fence around our house), and one man who brought us fresh fish off his deep sea trawler, which we credited at market value. He would come in as necessary and we'd take the charge off the credit he'd built up. Another man wanted to trade automotive work for care, and we went out to his shop, which turned out to look more like a junk yard than a shop with old rusting cars and junk all over the premises. We declined.

I had continued to barter with various patients and one young local dairy farmer brought his wife in for OB care asking if I would consider bartering for beef. Now with five kids of our own, I had no problem with that. As it happened she ended up requiring a C-section, and afterward he came in and asked what they owed. He would translate everything into sides of beef, and we got one each year. He raised one beef cow each year and gave us half and his family took half. They had two more children by C-section over the next few years, and his family and mine became good friends. He also supplied my garden with stuff from the dairy floor, which helped things grow very well.

I always reported the barter on my taxes because I felt we were in such a small area, the IRS local office might very well know the bartering and it really was part of my income. One day a lady came in to talk about OB care, and she asked me how I felt about the IRS. I told her I'd never made enough to really worry about them. It turned out she was an IRS agent, and she told me they had to be especially careful of doctors because a number of them had a grudge against the IRS. I had known this lady because I sang in several local choirs, and she played bassoon in some of the orchestras. We took her on as an OB patient and she did well.

I was called in the very early hours of the morning for one of our patients who was drunk and had missed the push-bar on a glass door and gone through the glass with her face. She was cut up pretty badly, and they wanted me to repair the facial lacerations. The "lady" was a professor at the local university and not the type one expected from a bar incident, but as I started putting local in to begin the repair, she proved she belonged with the bar crowd as she began screaming and cussing. She started calling me names, and that was about all I was going to take. I removed the drapes and my gloves and told her they had called me to fix her face, which was really pretty ugly with all the lacerations. I told her I'd gladly go back to my warm bed and leave her ugly if she persisted in name calling and cursing. She got the point, and we got back to work without the hysterics. The repairs went fine, and I told her once it healed we'd see if the scars would need revision by a plastic surgeon, but as far as I know, she never asked.

One of the banes of the primary care physician is drug seekers. There are really two types with some overlap between them. The first type is composed of the abusers who want pain meds and tranquilizers. The second group is made up of professionals who get the drugs for resale to addicts. They are primarily interested in opiates and especially Dilaudid. I asked one of my patients who I knew to be an undercover narc (which I learned when he put an automatic on the counter when he undressed for a physical) why they did this. He told me heroin addicts would pay $50 a pill for Dilaudid to use to in place of heroin. These people figured if they could get ten Dilaudid pills a week, they would do fine.

These people would usually come in on Friday afternoon when they knew we were ready to get the week over with. They would claim to be traveling and really needed their medication for their back or migraines or whatever. Usually they would show you a bottle from another physician to "prove" they were legitimate. I remember one in particular who had a large sheath knife on his belt. I decided I wasn't about to argue with him, so I gave him a prescription for ten Dilaudid. When he left the office, I looked in the parking lot and saw he was driving a pickup with a camper on the back. I called the pharmacist down the street and told him to be slow about filling it. I then called the police and gave them a description of the camper. By the time they got there, he was back in his camper, having filled the prescription. When they looked in the back window, he was just in the process of putting a needle in his arm and they hauled him off to jail.

One of the best planned drug-seeking cases was a man who claimed to be a psychologist visiting from Guam and having a terrible migraine. When I went into the exam room, he had turned off the lights and was holding his head. With the lights off and his hands over his face, it would be very hard to identify him, and with Guam twelve hours or so off from our time, I couldn't reach anyone to check on him. He was playing the colleague card to the hilt as a "fellow health-care professional." I turned the light on and took his hands away from his face, so I could check his pupils and see his face. I gave him his prescription and had the cops meet him as he came out the door of the pharmacy.

Since each department had to have backup for patients who didn't have their own physicians, I got called for a lady at term who had come in in labor. She had no real prenatal care and wanted anesthetic but violently refused needles. She hadn't been trained in Lamaze as most of my patients were, so about all I could offer her was hypnosis, which I told her might or might not work without training ahead of time. She wanted to try and was in fact able to maintain a trance for most of her labor with just a little re-enforcement from me. Her delivery went normally, and my status with the OB nurses went up about four notches.

There was an Indian reservation in the mountains about forty miles away, and we would get interesting trauma from there. One young man was brought in after a motorcycle accident. He was apparently on his way to a party with a case of beer on the back of his motorcycle when he hit an animal. The motorcycle had black hair on it, but the ambulance drivers weren't certain whether it came from a cow or a bear. Regardless, the cycle stopped abruptly, and the beer didn't. The case of beer drove his abdomen into the handlebars, and he had an acute abdomen. The surgeon and I took him into surgery where we found he had a fractured liver, which was bleeding heavily, especially when we took off the back pressure by opening the abdomen. As anyone who has handled beef liver will know, this is soft tissue. If you tie a suture in it too hard the suture itself will cut through making the bleeding worse. We would try to cauterize the vessels and used materials to encourage clotting (not nearly as good as are available now), but we never could get the bleeding under good control so the surgeon packed the abdomen with sterile towels and closed under pressure, which controlled the bleeding. We came back the next day and were able to remove the towels and close normally. Because of the massive trauma, the surgeon transferred him down to San Francisco where he did fairly well, but about the third day he developed shock lung (fluid in the lung from trauma) and died.

I was finishing a delivery in the hospital in the middle of the night when the ER called and said one of my patients was there asking for me. When I got there, I found a young Indian woman who had had a name I'd always been partial to. She had a last name that translated to "Young Running Crane." Unfortunately she'd married a Polish guy so that name was no more. When she'd gotten married, they had moved to the next town, and she was no longer coming to me. The story was that she'd gotten drunk and driven her car through a store front. She'd had some abdominal pain and been seen by one of the better surgeons in the area, but he'd decided she didn't need surgery at that time. Her mother was taking her to stay with her for the night, but by the time they got as far as our hospital her pain was getting much worse. When I examined her, I found that she had a surgical (rigid and extremely painful) abdomen. I told her she needed surgery now, and they decided they wanted to go back to the surgeon they'd seen earlier in the evening. I called him and told him what I found and that except for pain she seemed stable and he agreed to see her back. He called me the next day to tell me she died on the operating table. She had fractured her liver in the accident, but the liver capsule had remained intact so she did pretty well until the blood accumulating under the capsule caused enough pain. When they'd opened her abdomen, they could see what they had and prepared for the blood pressure drop they knew would happen when the capsule was opened, but when they opened it, the blood loss came so fast and the low pressure was so profound, they couldn't ever get control and she died. I felt very badly about her death, but secretly I was glad she'd elected to go back to the surgeon in the next town so we didn't have this disaster happen in our hospital.

Our new house was about ten miles north of the actual town, and we only had a volunteer fire department, which was self-financed mostly by a blackberry pie sale by the wives of the firefighters. They had an old 1936 Mack fire truck. We lived at the top of a hill, and they found they couldn't drive the truck up the hill because it had a gravity fuel system and no fuel pump. When they started up the hill, the engine would die, so they decided if they got called to our neighborhood, they'd back up the hill. Apparently this worked because they got to my neighbor's place when he had a chimney fire.

Because this fire department relied on the volunteers, they didn't happen to have any EMTS in the area and relied on the paramedics with the ambulance company in town when they had a medical call. The ambulance company was small, and sometimes the ambulance was tied up, so the fire chief approached me to ask if I would back them up. The deal was that if they couldn't get the ambulance to come immediately, they would call me, and if I was available, the chief would drive to my place and either lead me or take me to the emergency. The woods around there were full of small unmarked or poorly marked roads, so I was unlikely to find the call on my own.

The urgent calls we got were universally related to alcohol. The first such call involved a man who was so drunk he wouldn't respond, and although he looked OK, I had him sent to the hospital where he was admitted for alcohol poisoning. A week later we were called to the same address for a woman not breathing. When we arrived, we had to step over the same man to get to the back room where a very drunk young man had been performing mouth to mouth on a naked woman in the bed with him. I doubted he was very effective, but she seemed to be pink. When I watched her closely, she was breathing on her own but not well. We sent her into the hospital, and the ambulance crew told me later they had assisted her breathing because they weren't sure she was moving enough air.

We had another call that was very difficult to find, and when we did find the location we found an inebriated man sitting outside a travel trailer. He told us, "Ah'm just a swallerin' my tongue." He would then make choking sounds and repeat the phrase. He was obviously not in any distress but psychological and we just waited for the ambulance to transport him to the ER for evaluation. He told us he'd "swallered" his tongue once before when he lived in Las Vegas.

I had one family who were all mentally challenged. The father worked for a sheltered workshop and the mother didn't, as far as I know, ever work. One day they had scheduled a wart removal for their son, but when they came in, I noticed he had one eye held shut and tearing. I asked what had happened, and they told me another child had shot him in the eye with a paperclip and rubber band in school the previous day. When I got his eyelid open, I could see the pupil was not round and there was a puncture wound leaking fluid. I sent them straight to the ophthalmologist who took him to surgery. Normally the eye people helped each other in the OR, but this day they were all busy so he asked if I could assist. I was a little concerned because like most folks I was squeamish about the eye, but I went ahead and scrubbed in to help. Working through the operating microscope, we tried to clean up the iris, and after cleaning carefully, we were able to close the layers with the smallest suture I'd ever worked with. Just breathing around this stuff would send it floating away and the needle wasn't much heavier. We patched him up and he was admitted for a day or so. We did manage to save the eye, but he could barely see light and dark with it. The mother brought him back a couple months later, and we finally got his wart treated.

Sue and I were both active in adoption circles, and one day I got a call at the office about a baby who had been born in San Francisco with only one arm and no legs who had been scheduled for private adoption whose adoptive parents took a hike when they learned she wasn't perfect. When I got home that evening, I learned Sue had been called by another person about the same baby. We were intrigued and sat down as a family to discuss this. We had just completed a major remodel on our home so each of the kids would have a room of his or her own, but little Bridget volunteered to share her room with the baby. Sue was teaching at the local university, but felt since it was only half time, she could manage. We went ahead and called the birth mother and she seemed receptive. She was a nurse who had been accepted at medical school and the birth father was supportive but they had no intention of marrying. It was agreed that we could adopt the baby and the birth father drove the baby up to us at three days of age. We had intended to stop at four kids, but there didn't seem to be a huge difference with five. We already had a wheelchair ramp and we had a friend who had the same disability and was raising two boys by herself and doing just fine.

Our Ob-Gyn decided he would do better on his own because he feared he wasn't getting referrals from primary docs because they were afraid the patients would decide to stay with us. We were really relieved because he was so hard to deal with and sometimes made the office miserable. Since he was an owner, the financial negotiations were terrible, but finally successful and he left to open an office elsewhere in town.

We felt we'd be better off with another FP rather than try to recruit another OB, and among our applicants was one man who had changed fields. He had a PhD in theoretical math and had taught a short time at Cal Tech before going back to get his MD. He'd completed his residency in the Midwest and was ready to go into practice. He too became a mainstay of the practice.

I was called in to help the surgeon with a knife wound coming from the reservation. This was a single stab in the mid abdomen. The patient told us that in the midst of love making, he mistakenly called his wife by her sister's name. Apparently his wife slept with a knife under her pillow and she used it. When we started the surgery, we found the knife had gone through the stomach. As we freed the stomach from its attachments, we were getting into more and more bleeding. The general surgeon packed some towels into the abdomen and told the nurses to call the vascular and thoracic surgeon. I just stood there and controlled the bleeding until he arrived and stayed on to help him. We found the knife had penetrated the pancreatic artery and extended back into the right renal artery and vein. We were able to control the bleeding and start repairing vessels until we closed everything including the hole in the stomach. Post op the patient did fine and eventually left the hospital in good shape. I wouldn't be surprised if he became single shortly thereafter.

My next-door neighbor was a man in his eighties who was somewhat irascible and a bit difficult to live with. He had had problems with a duodenal diverticulum, which is a pouch from the bowel, which will get infected. Most diverticula are in the colon, but his was in the first portion of the small bowel coming out of the stomach. After he had a couple bouts of infection, we had put him on prophylactic antibiotics, which after a time he had quit taking. He began getting severe abdominal pain but refused to allow his wife to call anyone. So he was in pain all day until he passed out when she called an ambulance. When I saw him in the ER, an x-ray revealed free air in his abdomen, which meant the diverticulum had ruptured. Although I was very dubious about his chances, his wife wanted everything done so we took him to surgery. When the surgeon opened the peritoneum (lining of the abdomen), there was a hissing sound of gas escaping, and I had to tell myself to concentrate on what we were doing because if I thought about what I was smelling, I would lose it. Throwing up in a surgical mask is especially nasty. He'd been leaking digestive juices for hours and essentially was digesting his own abdominal contents externally. We closed the hole and rinsed the abdomen thoroughly to remove the enzymes and acid and closed the abdomen. Amazingly he survived in our ICU for two days, but eventually he was unable to continue and died.

One of the physicians at the Indian Clinic north of us invited us to go to a fund-raising picnic at the clinic. The menu consisted entirely of native foods. We thought this would be a great adventure and it was.

We tried the various foods such as elk, eel, acorn soup, salmon, and so on. I was very impressed with the eels, which surprised me by how good they were, but we had been warned that the acorn soup was an acquired taste and I must agree, it having all the allure of kindergarten paste. I asked why there was no venison and one of the organizers told us laughingly that they had to buy the venison because California's game laws would not let them use wild game, and the shipment was late. When they tracked the shipment, it was sitting in a warehouse in another town with a similar name. It had been sitting for two weeks without refrigeration, so the Indians never told them, figuring they would soon "smell" out the problem.

I was passing the ER one evening when the staff stopped me to ask if I could hang around as they had an ambulance coming in with three severely injured patients. When they arrived, there was a father and two children. One of the kids was in cardiac arrest, so I took that one and the other child while the ER physician took the adult who had severe injuries. The child they were trying to resuscitate was said to have been thrown from the pickup truck and was found face down in an icy creek. We worked with him for a little while, but it was quickly obvious there was nothing to work with so I turned my attention to the other child who had moderate hypothermia but otherwise seemed to have mostly bumps and bruises. We learned later that the first child had had a broken neck and probably died before the ambulance got there.

We ended up hiring another Ob-Gyn as our relations with the old one were somewhat strained and the only other one in town was a South Asian lady who was very nice, but our patients didn't care too much for her. She made a good portion of her income by doing abortions.

As I came to the hospital one day I saw the wife of our previous OB arrive in a taxi. She got out and walked to his Porsche (his pride and joy) and kicked in his grill. She then got back into the cab and drove off. They eventually got divorced, and I was happy it happened before someone got killed.

Out of nowhere Sue got pregnant again. We really hadn't expected this to happen after all the difficulties of her getting pregnant the first time, but everything went smoothly and Kathleen was born by repeat C-section. Now there were six, and it seemed time to stop.

Our woman physician decided she wanted to take an ER job and move to a town about 150 miles from us, so we started recruiting again. One of the applicants was a physician who was just completing his residency in Internal Medicine at Stanford. It turned out he had been the resident I had talked with when we transferred our patient with the super high temps there, and he was impressed with the completeness of our work-up. He'd been in the Public Health Service before his residency and had run a hospital on an isolated Indian reservation. While doing this, he'd grandfathered into taking the Family Practice boards and was boarded in Family Practice. New specialty boards will have a grandfather clause for a few years so physicians already practicing that specialty will have a chance to take the boards without attending residency. We felt this would be a good fit and he took his Internal Medicine Boards and joined us double boarded. He became one of the mainstays of our group.

I was asked by one of my patients if I would consider becoming an FAA medical examiner so I could do physicals for private pilots. I looked into it and the requirements were fairly easy except we needed one or two additional eye exam pieces of equipment. We got those, and then my medical assistant and I went to a course the FAA held. I was impressed that they were really concerned that we get the forms filled out right and said very little about the exam itself. The next step up was to become a flight surgeon, but that required the purchase of a very expensive ECG transmitter and there already was one flight surgeon in our area. The only difference was the ability to certify level one licenses, which are for scheduled commercial airline pilots.

After we got started, we began to get a steady group of pilots needing physicals, and I began to realize they were pretty liberal with their rules. One young man wanted to get his pilot's license but had had a heart transplant. I did his exam but kicked the final determination upstairs to the regional flight surgeon. He cleared the young man pointing out that he had a myocardial biopsy every month and was watched much more closely than our other pilots.

Another young man came in, and my medical assistant warned me this wasn't going to be easy. This patient was sixteen, which was the minimum age, and told me he had always wanted to be a pilot. He had a heart defect that let some un-oxygenated blood cross to the systemic side without going through the lungs. This resulted in a chronic bluish tint and obvious slight shortness of breath. In addition, the defect had had a clot form, which went to his brain, causing a septic stroke (stroke with a brain abscess), and he was partially paralyzed. I did his exam but had to tell him I didn't think he could pass because he was short of breath at sea level, and there was no way he could go to altitude. Again I kicked it up to the regional flight surgeon and he agreed. I felt bad having to explain to this young man that the thing he most wanted to do in this world he couldn't do. It seems people with disabilities at that age often try to deny their problem and need to be forced to look realistically at what they can and can't do. Young diabetics are notorious for trying to ignore their problem.

We were also doing physicals for a couple of local trucking companies. For some licenses the state required physicals, and the companies would pay for them. One man came in on the day after Labor Day about ten in the morning. He knew he would be drug tested. When I did his exam, he smelled strongly of alcohol. He also told me he had a DUI on his record. After the exam I called the company and advised them he was not someone they wanted driving an eighteen wheeler, and they agreed. He turned up in my waiting room shouting that I had ruined his life, and I was so angry I met him nose to nose and told him in front of everyone that he wasn't driving a big truck if he couldn't even come in for an exam sober. He claimed it was because he had been playing softball on Labor Day and *had* to drink beer. It takes a lot of beer for you to still be drunk at 10:00 a.m. the next day.

The drug testing we had to do was interesting. The law in California wouldn't let us observe the patient getting the specimen, so they would go into the rest room and get their specimen and bring it out where our lab tech would immediately take the temperature of the urine. We had a couple fellows who were trying to keep their girlfriends' urine warm in their pocket, and the bottle leaked leaving them with a large wet spot on their pants. Another smart-aleck had hand warmers in his pocket with the urine and had a temp of 107, which we didn't buy. We did have to set a lower limit on cannabis because the test is so sensitive it would show secondary exposure and exposure from a month or more previous. Our employers were interested in levels that showed recent or chronic usage so we told the lab not to report levels lower than 50 ppm.

Around this time we were contacted by a dermatologist who was finishing his training at UCLA and was looking for a place to practice. He and his wife came up and interviewed and turned out to be nice people with whom one of the partners hit it off with very well. Since there was no dermatologist in town, we decided to take a chance and hire him. He went back to southern California to finish his last month or two. The next thing I heard was a call from him saying he was in jail in Los Angeles. It was never very clear why, but he wanted us to send him a small amount of money to bail him out. We did with great trepidation, and soon he called back to say he'd had some sort of psychological upset. I told him we couldn't have that sort of thing happening in a small town, and he agreed to have his psychiatrist call and talk to me. This man claimed it was just the pressure of finishing up and would be a one-time occurrence. He assured me we didn't have to worry about recurrence. We went ahead and kept him on.

Our new dermatologist was very well liked and seemed to be busy. He had one dislike, however, and that was crab lice. Of all the ugly skin diseases available, this one bothered him, and apparently he was seeing quite a few cases. It didn't take long for the office assistants to figure this out. One of the women worked weekends as a cocktail waitress at a local restaurant and got hold of some rubber Dungeness crabs they used for display. At the end of the day his last chart had the complaint of "another case of crabs." When he went into the room after a little grumbling, he found a wooden case with the rubber crabs arranged around it on the exam table. He seemed to enjoy the joke.

Often we'd get bored with seeing colds about which we could do very little, but one lady got our attention after she came to see me with a severe sore throat. Since her strep screen was negative, I told her it just looked like a viral sore throat. She came back in with the same sore throat and saw our internist. He came to the same conclusion as

I had, but four days later she was back. Now she had added a strange rash. The internist decided to get additional lab work and took her down the hall to our lab. She passed our new dermatologist in the hall, and he called the internist over to tell him the rash looked like a leukemic rash. Shortly thereafter we discovered our Coulter Counter (the machine that does blood counts) turned out to have lights we didn't even know were there. As the white count rolled past a hundred thousand a little light lit up, and before it was done there were four little lights lit. This meant she had a white count of over four hundred thousand when normal is less than ten thousand. We called her back in and put her in the hospital while we got a bone marrow and arranged to transfer her to Stanford. We made the diagnosis on a Tuesday and flew her to Stanford on Wednesday. They called us and said with this type of leukemia the best they'd ever managed was to keep the patient alive for six months and that required such a nasty chemo regimen that the patients were miserable the whole time. They were going to phorese her blood to remove the huge number of white cells for fear that the blood would be so thick it would clot. In fact on her way to the procedure she had a stroke and died, which I thought probably was better than prolonged suffering.

Fortunately I was not on call the night the police called our on-call doc about the dermatologist. They had been called by his neighbors about him running a chainsaw in the middle of the night. It turned out he was "remodeling" his house by cutting out the windows with a chainsaw. His wife and children had fled, and he made comments he wanted to kill them. My partner who was on-call helped get him calmed down, and he was taken to the locked psychiatric facility. The previous episode was now explained. He was a manic-depressive and he'd just gone manic. His psychiatrist in LA had lied to me about this being a single incident, which would not recur.

About a week later I was alone in the office at lunch hour when he came in the door at the end of the far wing. I thought it might be all over when I saw he was wearing a holster, but when he got closer, I could see he had a hairbrush in the holster. I've never before been delighted to see a hairbrush. He told me he was on medications and needed to get a Lithium level. Lithium was one of the few direct treatments for manic-depressive syndrome but needed to be monitored very carefully because the therapeutic range is very close to the toxic range. I told him the lab should be back from lunch very soon and went back to my charts. I heard him in the lab and went in to see what he was doing. I found him with a tourniquet on his arm, which he was holding with his teeth like an addict, while he tried to draw his own blood. Apparently his control wasn't all that good yet.

Naturally we had to let him go since the entire town knew the story or soon would. His wife moved to Canada where part of her family was, and we never heard about her or the children again. We got requests for references from several medical groups in the Bay Area, and I had to be completely honest that he was a good dermatologist but would have to be monitored to make sure he stayed on his medications. We heard later he had been hired at one of those groups but apparently went into a deep depression and committed suicide, an unfortunate outcome of a terrible disease.

From the time I started doing deliveries in medical school, the fastest changing field in medicine seemed to be OB. Interestingly it seemed somewhat schizophrenic with the patients wanting rooms that didn't look high-tech and wanting nurse midwives while the field was going much higher tech with electronic monitors and suction forceps (a plumbers friend for the baby's head) as well as intrauterine blood pH monitoring, to say nothing of amniotic fluid sampling and ultrasound. This high tech versus low tech caused problems. I had hired the first nurse midwife in our hospital, and she was very popular with the patients because she was able to spend more time with them and would always deliver her own patients. As time went on, however, she seemed to become less and less sure of herself and called me worried about the monitor patterns on almost every delivery. It began to seem more difficult to have her working than to just do it myself. As all these technical changes came in, the expected results were changed. When I was in medical school, we were told the still birth rate would be about 5 percent and the C-section rate would be about 5 percent as well. By the time I was well into practice, the C-section rate gradually increased to about 20 percent. Meanwhile, if you delivered a still birth you would be called before the OB committee to explain yourself.

We had put in two alternative birth rooms, but these were really just fluff. There were hidden stirrups and packs of forceps etc. hidden in a room with a full bed and lacy curtains. The husbands and often the whole family would attend and I would have to warn the husbands not to use flash cameras during the delivery so I wouldn't be blinded. They had music systems to play, and I told my partners that one lady sounded like she wanted the whole Mormon Tabernacle Choir to sing the "Hallelujah" chorus while she delivered, and I had to explain the room was only so large.

As these changes were pushed in the training centers, some of the older methods ceased to be taught. I had had to learn to do rotational forceps as well as outlet forceps, premature forceps and Piper forceps for breeches as part of my residency. We would get young Ob-Gyns who wanted to practice in our area who didn't know how to do any of those things. When I was chief of the OB committee, I would ask them what they would do if the baby's heart rate fell to below sixty beats per minute and stayed there. They would always answer they would go to the delivery room and do a C-section. I had to explain the fastest we could do one was twenty minutes, and at night it was considerably longer. We had two OR crews, an anesthesiologist with only part of his residency, and a nurse anesthetist. Only one team was on call each night, and they had to come from home. Each night before they left, they set up for a C-section but it still took a little time and therefore you needed to be looking far ahead and to be able to use such things as forceps to get out of trouble. I was told by one university type we shouldn't be doing OB if we couldn't have the OB suite staffed to do C-sections. I asked him if he really thought the patients from our area should travel about two hundred miles for their care.

Sometimes we ran into ethical dilemmas. One patient called to tell me he had gotten plane tickets to his daughter's graduation from college back east but had changed his plans and wanted me to write a letter to the airline stating he was sick and had to cancel his flight. I pointed out this wasn't true and constituted fraud and refused to help. He was very angry, and we never saw him as a patient again.

That same patient had gotten a divorce, and I hadn't seen his wife for a while when she came in looking terrible. She said she was running out of things to eat. The story was that she'd met a man who claimed to be an allergist. He actually lived in Nevada and flew in to see patients for a day or two and flew out again. He had a machine he claimed was from Europe and that American physicians didn't know about. This machine had two handles, which the patient was supposed to hold, and the machine would tell him which foods they had allergies to. This lady was down to broccoli as the only food she was allowed to eat.

I asked where he had his office, and she admitted she allowed him to use her home. I was in a quandary that this was patient information and should be confidential, but also this was criminal activity and, I was convinced, could very well kill her. I went ahead and notified the district attorney's office of this obvious medical scam, and they shut him down. I also lost the other half of this couple as a patient.

Sometimes patients completely surprise you. I had a lady whom I knew to be a member of a strict religion who came in with a strange story. Her husband had died a year or so before, and she told me she was finally over grieving and wished to return to life, so she took a cruise up the coast of Alaska. On the ship she met three men and moved into their cabin. She said they really didn't see the tour because they seldom left the cabin. She had been penetrated in every orifice and now felt terrible. When I examined her, she had a purplish rash and fever as well as discharge from the vagina, rectum, and exudate in her throat. It was apparent she had gonococcemia (gonorrhea in the blood stream), which can be very dangerous. I confirmed the diagnosis in the lab and advised her she needed to be in the hospital. In spite of my best arguments, she adamantly refused hospitalization because she was sure the story would get out, and she'd lose her job as a teacher in a religious school. The best I could get was her promise that she would let me admit her if she didn't respond to antibiotics readily. We started her on mega doses of antibiotics and I saw her the next day. She was a little better the following day, so we continued the antibiotic regimen and continued to follow her daily as she slowly got better. Just shows that even a matronly school teacher may have secrets.

I never ceased to be amazed that intelligent college-educated people could do amazingly stupid things. One man came in with complaints that were obviously nervous in origin, and I asked him what was causing him stress. He told me his wife had moved her boyfriend into their house. He was trying to be very sophisticated about the whole thing but really was as angry as most people would be. When I told him he needed a good divorce lawyer and he needed to throw both of them out of his house, he did those things and his anxiety went away.

As our group was becoming larger and better known, we were able to swing contracts for more work. One of the earlier ones was with the coast guard. They had three facilities in our area: a small boat rescue group, a coast guard cutter, and at the nearby airfield, a rescue helicopter unit. The coast guard doesn't have their own physicians but can use the military facilities and the units in our area could go to the naval hospital in Oakland but it was several hours away and not convenient. Therefore they preferred to have routine things done by us locally. This also meant we got more of the OB cases those young people were generating.

One of the jobs we did for the coast guard was reenlistment physicals. I was very familiar with the forms as they were the same as those used by the air force. I had an old chief come in for his re-enlistment exam, and he told me he had been in the navy first then transferred to the coast guard. Like many of the older navy-enlisted personnel, he was covered with tattoos. The medical exam form wanted descriptions of all distinguishing marks, I assume for body identification in case of crash. It took me over an hour to describe his tattoos and he agreed if he needed to re-enlist again, he'd get it done at a military facility.

One eighteen-year-old coast guardsman came in with a cold. I was listening to his lungs when I noted the scariest skin lesion I'd seen at that point in practice. I told him we needed to remove the lesion that day and he agreed. I excised the lesion with some margin and sent it for pathology. The report came back that it was a superficial spreading melanoma. We contacted dermatology at the naval hospital, but they couldn't see him for two months. That was longer than seemed reasonable to me, so I scheduled him for re-excision and took an additional 2 cm around the original lesion. Fortunately this was on his back so the resulting scar wasn't visible. He did get to dermatology eventually, and they agreed with my treatment and set up to follow him for recurrence since even with aggressive margins, about 20 percent of these will come back. He remained in our area for about a year and still was doing well when he was transferred to another duty station. He later told me that when I told him it needed to be removed immediately, he thought I was padding the coast guard's bill.

The coast guard commander called to set up appointments for a pilot and copilot who had crashed one of the rescue helicopters. They required a physical and psychological evaluation after an accident before the pilot could go back to flying, just as the air force had. When they came in, the pilot told me they had been involved in a rescue just off the coast in rough waters. Their diver was down in the water saving a fisherman who had capsized, and they were all watching through the open door while they hovered over the scene. Unfortunately they didn't see a rogue wave, which must have been thirty feet high when it hit the chopper and took them down. The pilot said when these choppers hit the water they would immediately turn upside down. He said they had practiced getting out of their belts and escaping the cabin in a pool so often he just did it automatically and didn't realize what had happened until he was on the surface. They were all rescued by the other helicopter they had at the base. The only good thing that came out of it was they got a brand-new helicopter, which they'd needed for some time. The taxpayer, however, lost $3 million.

We got a call one day from the coast guard that they had picked up a man from a Russian trawler off the coast who may have had appendicitis. They flew him to the hospital by helicopter, and when he was seen, he turned out to be a Siberian who spoke no English. His exam was indeed very suspicious for appendicitis, and although we had no interpreters, we were able to get him to understand that he needed surgery. In the OR he was found not to have appendicitis but did have holes in his cecum and numerous little worms crawling around in his abdomen. The surgeon washed out the worms and closed the holes. We had no idea what these things were but they were sent to the parasitologist at the local university who gave them to the wildlife parasitologist. He was able to identify them as a worm of pinnipeds, which are seals, sea lions, and walruses. These critters go through a phase in a fish and then go into the fish's muscle where they get released when the fish is eaten by a pinniped. They are then supposed to live in the gut and pass eggs out with the pinniped's feces and back into the sea. This man had apparently been eating raw fish on the trawler, and when the worms got into his gut, they got confused and became a problem. He recovered nicely and was taken back to his ship.

I understand these same worms can turn up in sushi and Japanese sushi chefs are trained to recognize them.

We were contacted by a local lumber company to do some industrial work for them. They had a couple of lumber mills and a couple of plywood mills as well in the area. We went with their safety director to tour both types of facility, so we'd know what the jobs were. He was going to take us into the woods as well, but we never got there although I had a pretty good idea what those jobs entailed having watched the lumberjacks work when I was cutting firewood. The mills were pretty scary because they seemed to have been designed by engineers without allowing for the people working there. For example, in the lumber mill you could only get from one side to the other by ducking under active belts carrying wood. First the logs went into a device called the de-barker and were tumbled around while being hit with a very high pressure water hose, which removed the bark. Some of the bark was sold to gardeners and the rest was burned to supply electricity to run the mill.

The logs were then sliced into boards by giant saws, and the boards were taken down a chain where a man decided what lengths would give the most boards. He had a keyboard like a typewriter, which would raise or lower a series of saws to cut lengths. The boards then went to the "green chain" where the green lumber was separated by length and thickness and stacked by hand. Since it was still green, it was very heavy, and over the years, we saw a lot of back and other problems from the men and women on the green chain. They were paid by production and worked as a team, so if someone wasn't keeping up, they cost everybody money, which was a great incentive not to slack off.

One of the first exams I did for the company was a little Native American who had a pretty big beer belly. He had been laid off for a couple of years and was about to restart, but the company questioned whether he was in good-enough shape to do his job. He was a choker setter, which meant he would drag heavy cables around the logs that had been cut so they could be dragged out of the woods. This required running and jumping over logs while pulling the heavy choker cable. The patient told me to stay in shape he had been running two miles daily since he was laid off. His physical was normal as was his ECG, but I decided to put him through a treadmill test to see if he could tolerate such stress. He actually completed stage 6 on the Bruce scale, the equivalent of running up a long, steep hill. I told the company that in spite of appearances, he was capable of doing the job, and he happily went back to work.

The company had had a policy that if a man couldn't do his regular job, he was to be put on disability. They began to find that their disability insurance was getting too expensive and made a complete reversal that if the employee could do anything, he was to be returned to the company and they'd find him work. Shortly after this change, a man came in with a badly sprained ankle. I examined this and sent him back with a note that he could not bear weight on that ankle for the next two weeks. He came back for follow-up and I was curious what they'd done with him. He told me they'd put him to work painting all the baseboards in the company offices so he could just crawl around all day.

An electrician from the plywood plant was sent to me for evaluation. He had recently been diagnosed with epilepsy and was on heavy doses of medication. His job involved repairing the motors on cranes near the four-story ceiling. These motors were on the ends of long arms, and to get to them, he had to walk out the arm on a catwalk, which was about eighteen inches wide and had no railings. When I saw him, he was moving very slowly and with poor coordination secondary to his medications (it's called ataxia). I told the company that if he continued on his present medications, he would be unsafe if he had to work on anything above the floor of the plant and indeed he shouldn't get close to the hot presses used to glue the plywood panels together. They told me they had a job he could do with those restrictions and receive the same pay. I heard however that the union objected to changing his job description and threatened to strike if his job was changed. They called his physician who certified he was safe without ever seeing what he did, and the company was forced to keep him in the same job although the foreman said he would not let him climb. It was the first of many times when I felt the union was more interested in their power than in the employee's safety. Because the company had liability, they were very concerned about safety.

The safety director at the company was also one of our regular patients, and he told me one day that he had invented a safety device to be used in the woods. As described previously, a common injury with chain saws occurred when the faller or lumberjack rested the saw on their anterior thigh. Fairly regularly they would do this before the chain had stopped moving even though they had taken their finger off the trigger. This would result in a nasty laceration and take the man out of work for several weeks. The safety director decided to try to see if Kevlar (the material used in bullet-proof vests) would stop the chain before injury occurred. He found that seven layers would indeed stop the chain as long as the trigger wasn't engaged. He had chaps made up for the men, but they refused to wear them. He had to have these made to fit into their jeans so the other men couldn't see they were wearing them and tease them about being sissies.

I discovered one of my partners was color-blind. He had always been the butt of some of the office girl's jokes because of his wardrobe, but I had not realized what at least part of the problem was until one day when he and I were the only ones in the office and we got a call from the local university. They told us they had a water-polo match that evening, and the team had not yet had the required physicals. The AAU required these before they could play and the game could be official. They had planned on getting them done at the Student Health Unit, but their power had gone down and they couldn't do them. We agreed to stay after work and get them done. When the athletes arrived, I told my partner I'd take one wing of the building and do half, and he could do the other half in the other wing. One requirement on the form was an Ishihara colorblindness test. I could not understand why they cared, but I suppose the form was for every college sport and it might matter in some. I was working away when my partner called me to ask if I'd do his Ishiharas. I was a bit irritated until he told me he didn't know when they were correct because he was totally colorblind himself.

While doing these physicals, I noted one player had a history of several fractures and his exam revealed that the whites of his eyes were bluish. When I asked, he admitted he had *osteogenisis imperfecta,* which is a congenital disorder with weak bones. He said this was the only sport he'd been able to play and pleaded with me to clear him. Since he'd played for several years and didn't have anything likely to be life-threatening, I cleared him but let the school know that he could be subject to fractures.

One of the duties of a small-town physician is helping out with the high school athletic program. In the state of California, there was a law that no varsity football game could be played without a physician in attendance. I felt it strange that the school nurse was good enough for the junior varsity games however. Indeed the worst injury I ever encountered on the football field occurred in a junior varsity game. I was just getting out of my car in the parking lot just behind the stands when I heard a loud "crack" coming from the field. I quickly went to the field where the side judge was lying in agony. The kids had run a play known as "student body right" where the ball carrier and about half the line try to get around the end of the line. When the carrier was pushed out of bounds, the judge had planted his foot to mark where the ball had gone out of bounds. Unfortunately both teams were still running, and one kid hit his leg high and another simultaneously hit the same leg low. The crack I heard was all the ligaments in his knee breaking simultaneously. We splinted him up and shipped him off in the ambulance to the ER and a future of a lot of surgery.

I would sit on the bench with the kids because they would try to hide their injuries, and I could better assess them. One time I was sitting there watching as the offense came off and heard the quarterback mumbling something. It turned out he was mumbling, "I can't remember the plays." I reassured him he didn't have to and informed the coach he was concussed and was out for the rest of the game.

At another game one young man stayed down after the play, and I went onto the field to check him. He'd hurt his shoulder, and after examining him (feeling under the pads), I concluded he had fractured his collarbone. This is a common injury and not terribly serious, so when he asked if he could sit on the bench and watch the rest of the game, I agreed. In a few moments his mother came out of the stands and wanted to take him to the ER. I told her there was no rush, and she said, "You don't understand that he's got hemophilia and needs treatment urgently." I was absolutely floored as all these kids were supposed to have been screened for health problems. It turned out I was backup for the ER that night, so they paged me when he got there because the ER doc didn't know what to do. By that time the game was over, and I went to the ER to check him.

In the ER he looked just fine, and I couldn't find any evidence of bleeding. I called his hematologist in San Francisco, and he felt we probably should give him a unit of factor eight anyway. I was concerned because AIDS was starting to rage in the area, and it takes several units of blood to provide one unit of factor eight. However, the hematologist told me the factor eight had not been safe and every one of his hemophilia patients in the Bay Area had AIDS but with a new heat treatment it was again safe to use.

The factor eight arrived from our local blood bank, and before the nurses hung the bag, I asked to see it. I could not find any place where it said it had been heat treated. I called the hematologist back, and he confirmed it should be prominently marked on the unit. When I called the blood bank, they admitted this was an older unit and sent a current one clearly marked as heat treated. Things went fine for the boy although I pulled him out of football, and the next day the chief of the blood bank and I had some words. I pointed out that not throwing this unit out to save money could have been a death sentence for this kid, and they changed their policies.

As time progressed, I was becoming more involved in the administrative aspects of medicine. I was invited to join the board of directors of the Consortium for Medical Care for the county and began to see what was going on in some other offices in my area. The consortium was really a billing agency for Blue Cross and other insurance carriers. The board was used primarily to decide if a bill was appropriate when it was questioned. We had one solo lady practitioner who was very inclined to double bill patients for such things as ECGs, which she would do in her office, even though she had already done one in the hospital and the patient's status had not changed. She got very upset when we started disallowing these. There were a number of physicians who tended to have questionable billing tactics, and we were sometimes able to teach appropriate billing practices.

Because our office was so involved in doing occupational medicine I was contacted by the local medical society because they had a request from the state medical society for a representative to the state Industrial Medicine Committee. It didn't seem to involve a lot of time, so I agreed. Since the committee was statewide we met by telephone conference and only had one face to face meeting in the time I was a member. This was held at the Airport Hilton in San Francisco which was a fairly central location.

At the meeting I felt really out of place as the other members were all dressed in what appeared to be tailor-made suits and were wearing Rolexes. I was the only country doc in the bunch and looked it with my J. C. Penny's sport coat and Timex. The biggest thing on the agenda was a group in Southern California who were charging $6,000 for a disability work-up whereas these guys were all charging about $4,000. I had never charged more than $400 and usually less for this workup. Maybe that's why my accountant kept asking why I didn't make as much as the other docs he did taxes for. I left that committee as soon as I reasonably could.

I was also asked to join the board of the county medical society. We had to deal with credentialing problems as well as impaired physicians. Alcoholism is always a problem in high-stress fields, and medicine is no exception. We also tried to plan ahead for county medical needs. One problem that was never resolved was that we had four hospitals in an area with less than a hundred thousand population. The result was that they all were small, and they all were lacking in equipment because no single hospital could afford some of the most modern equipment and they really resisted co-operation.

Our former Ob-Gyn was becoming more and more explosive as time went on. Finally he had a screaming fit when one of his patients who was post-op from a vaginal hysterectomy had some heavy bleeding. It was apparent that a stitch had given way, but he couldn't accept that and wanted her room searched for the "douche stick" he swore she had to have been using. The lady went into hysterics and asked for another physician, which seemed reasonable. The Ob-Gyn was called before the medical board, which I was on, and he told us unless they backed him on this he was leaving. The next day every doc he met asked him where he was going. He was so amazed and embarrassed that he did indeed have to close shop and leave the area, much to everyone's relief.

Back in the office, I had a thirty-seven-year-old man who came in for a general physical who said he had noticed a lump and was curious what it was. I could feel a rock-hard lump in his right upper arm at the edge of the biceps muscle. This was under the skin and fat and about a centimeter in diameter. I advised him that I didn't know what it was, but if it weren't so hard I would think of a lipoma (a benign tumor of fat). I suggested that it should be biopsied but he wanted to think about it.

About two months later he came in and said he'd decided to go ahead with the biopsy because he thought it was growing a little. At the biopsy I was very concerned because this very hard blackish lump had a smaller similar lump next to it. Benign lumps seldom have babies. The pathology came back as a liposarcoma, which is a highly malignant tumor. I contacted an orthopedic surgeon at UC San Francisco who specialized in soft tissue tumors, and he agreed to see the patient. This surgeon took the patient back to surgery and cleaned out all the subcutaneous tissue and muscle fascia in the area after which the entire shoulder area was given radiation treatments. The patient came back for me to follow, which proved not to be easy since the radiation caused his lymph nodes in his arm pit to swell, and I had to biopsy several of them to be sure his tumor was not re-growing. He did fine and had no evidence of recurrence for the several years I continued to follow him.

The patient whose first baby was born without an intact diaphragm was pregnant again and delivered a normal little girl. About two years later I got an urgent call from the hospital that this child had been brought in with a severe head injury, and the family wanted me to come. The story was that the child had been playing in the yard when an elderly couple who lived next door were going somewhere and came out to get in their car. The child knew them as they were sort of surrogate grandparents and ran over to them. They didn't see her, and before her mother could get there, they had backed over the child. To make matters worse when they realized the child was under the car they drove forward running over her again.

When I got to the ER, the child was in shock and had signs of severe brain injury. The abdomen was swelling rapidly, and there was apparently hemorrhage there, which was going to kill her, so we went to the OR and found and removed a ruptured spleen. I then arranged transport to the next town where the only neurosurgeon was and followed them over. The neurosurgeon met us and arranged a CT scan, which showed very severe brain damage, and he felt there was nothing he could do. My pediatric consultant met us, and we sat down with the parents to decide what to do. After discussion the parents decided to have us remove the life support, which we did, and the parents and I stood and watched this baby die.

This mother eventually started a support group for parents who had a baby die and indeed got pregnant again and had a normal child by her third C-section. I told her that though it was recommended that we limit a patient to three C-sections, I would be willing to do a fourth for her because I was worried she would become overly protective, but she handled things well and I ended up referring an occasional patient to her group.

The hospital had a program where all the internists shared the duty of reading ECGs and monitoring treadmills. The internists billed for these services and made about $5,000 each month they were on duty. Our new internist applied for this privilege but was denied. We had patiently waited for over a year, and the hospital and other internists were still adamant that they wouldn't let him into the rotation. He had a friend in San Francisco who was a lawyer in a large firm, and he wrote him regarding this situation. His friend wrote back saying that this was an interesting restraint of trade case, and under the law, if we sued the hospital, the result would be three times the damages we had sustained by their denial of privileges. We sent a copy of the letter to the other internists and the hospital administration. The other internists just laughed it off, but when the hospital lawyer saw what firm was involved, he advised the hospital to put our doc on the rotation immediately, which they did.

I got a call from a mother of a teenager one day saying he had been rapidly losing weight and had developed a huge thirst. Her description made it obvious he was a new onset type 1 diabetic, and I told her we would have to get him in immediately and probably he would be hospitalized for a short time. She broke down in tears saying her husband was laid off (as were many at that time), and they couldn't afford the costs. I had her bring him down to the office and told her I wouldn't charge because I was so worried that he get immediate care. When they came in, his blood sugar was indeed very high. I told her we should hospitalize him, but I'd keep it to a minimum and that's what we did. He was admitted, started on insulin, and given IV fluids, and we had him in much better shape by the following day when I discharged him to be followed through the office. This family wasn't eligible for Medi-Cal because they owned their own house. The husband had always worked and they would have been required to sell their house to become eligible. I never understood that law and never felt it was fair.

Many people try to ignore the fact that medicine is a business, but if the practitioner does he'll be bankrupt in very little time. Unfortunately many people also believe the doctor is rich and really doesn't need the money, so they'll try to skip paying their medical bills. We had to become experts at collecting our bills and occasionally had to turn bills over to a collection agency. The man at the agency got half of what they collected, so we weren't wild about turning accounts over unless we'd exhausted all avenues.

One account we had to handle was a truck driver who we took to small claims court. He claimed he was laid off and had no money. The court found for us, and I told the man to let us know when he was back at work and we'd just have to wait. It happened that his boss's wife worked at the hospital, and one day I asked when he might bring back his drivers. She said her husband had worked hard to get enough work to keep his men going and hadn't laid off any drivers. I then asked what day he paid payroll. Armed with that information and the judgment, we looked through our records and found an old check he had given us. From that we had his checking account number, and we gave the county constable the account and asked he get our judgment on the day after payday. This he did and we collected our money. The man turned up a couple days later very angry because all his checks had bounced. I told him I was willing to help a guy out when he was down, but I really didn't like liars and had no sympathy for him.

We had one family that owned a popular Mexican restaurant who seemed to be doing pretty well, but they never paid their bills. We finally took them to small claims court and got a judgment. Many people seem to think there are no teeth in these judgments, but if you know what you're doing, there are lot of ways to enforce them. In this case they did not make any effort to meet their obligations, so we went back to court and the judge found in our favor. We then went to the constable and asked for a "till tap." We specified ten on Friday night. At that time the constable went to the restaurant with the court order and took all the money in the till, which still didn't meet the total of their bill, but they showed up at the office on Monday to pay the rest so they wouldn't be embarrassed again.

One of my friends was a college professor who was an expert in diseases of wildlife. One year on his physical I noted some white spots on his lower lip. Because he was a pipe smoker, I became concerned and did a Pap smear of the area. The smear came back compatible with leukoplakia, which is a pre-cancerous condition caused by the chronic irritation from by his pipe. I strongly encouraged him to quit smoking and suggested we get the plastic surgeon to do a procedure called a lip shave to make sure there wasn't already an area that had progressed to cancer. He really didn't want to go and asked if I could do it instead. I had read what the procedure consisted of and felt it really wasn't difficult, so after some negotiation I finally agreed to do it with the understanding that I hadn't done it before and he might end up wanting a plastic revision if it didn't come out as expected. The procedure itself consists of making an incision along the lip line and another at the mucosal junction. The skin of the lip is removed and the intraoral mucosa is advanced to the skin line. The books said this would convert itself into normal lip epidermis and indeed it did. His lip epidermis did show early changes but we got all of them and his lip healed so well that later I could not see what had been done, even knowing where the lines should have been.

My mathematician partner had decided to start a family and had asked if I would deliver their baby, which was flattering, and I did so. When they decided to have a second, his wife was due around Christmas. This was an important holiday for me with so many kids. We usually spent all morning with the kids opening a huge stack of presents from us and both sets of grandparents. On Christmas morning, the phone rang at around 6:00 a.m., and the nurses in OB said my partner and his wife were in, and she was going quickly. I was pretty disappointed, but I went in to find she was about to crown. I just had time to glove and gown when she gave a push and out came the baby. Everybody was fine, and I was back home by seven-thirty. I told them they could have as many babies as they wanted if they were always as quick as that.

Christmas could be problematic for us. There was a period of three years in a row when the vascular surgeon and I spent Christmas Eve in the OR doing carotid enarterectomies. These had all presented with evidence of near obstruction or clots, and we were afraid to make them wait over the holiday. The procedure consists of dissecting out the carotid artery and placing clamps or ties above and below the area of the arteriosclerosis. This was right near the bifurcation between the internal and external carotid and was probably caused by the turbulent flow. If it appeared simple and the brain had good blood flow from the other side on the arteriograms, we could just clamp and operate rapidly. If the removal of the plaque and closure of the artery took less than five minutes, you could get away without a shunt. If things looked difficult or the blood supply from the other side didn't look adequate, we would put a shunt in, bypassing the area we needed to clean out, and we could then take our time. If we could avoid clots (and therefore strokes), the post-op period was usually pretty simple since the procedure was really pretty superficial.

As time went by, we were approached by a woman with a master's degree in family counseling. Since this seemed a fit with our group, we provided her with office space and clerical help for a percentage, and things seemed to work out well. One day she came to me and asked if I would hold a gun for her. It seemed a client came in with this gun-threatening suicide. She persuaded him to give it up, and because she was afraid to store it, I took it home. After a few months he apparently was better and got his gun back.

Our local orthopedic surgeon was one of the best I had ever worked with. He had been a missionary doc before going back to his ortho residency, so he understood general medicine better than most. In addition he had an uncanny feel for what was under the area he was working on. He was so sure of where his screws and pins went he would start putting the cast on post-op before the x-rays were developed, and in all the time I worked with him, we only had to go back and adjust one screw. He was eventually so busy he decided to bring in a partner. His new partner came from his old residency but turned out to be an entirely different kettle of fish. In those days a knee meniscus was a big operation, which involved coming into the knee from the medial (toward the middle of the body) compartment and removing both menisci with a smaller incision over the lateral side and using a special instrument with a sharpened end to free the meniscus. I was helping the new partner when he seemed to lose it and couldn't decide whether he had the meniscus free or not and was afraid to cut it loose. It must have taken fifteen minutes before I convinced him he had the right tissue and got him to cut it.

Today of course the meniscus is done through the arthroscope and is repaired or trimmed of torn tissue but not usually removed in its entirety. The meniscus never regenerated very well anyway, and the recovery was slow, requiring about six months of rehab to restore function to the knee. Although we used the scopes in gynecological surgery only more recently have the general surgeons developed laparoscopic procedures for elsewhere in the abdomen such as the gallbladder and appendix. Likewise the orthopedic surgeons do much of their surgery with scopes today.

When I was in the air force, pilots with ulcers were required to have a procedure called a vagotomy and pyloroplasty, which caused the stomach to make less acid and to have a larger opening to the small bowel. During my years of private practice I assisted dozens of such procedures for ulcers, which didn't always work well. Now we know that most ulcers are caused by *Helicobactor pylori*, a bacterium that lives in the stomach. All those people had unnecessary surgery if we had only known. I suspect most surgical residents aren't really well trained today in what was a bread-and-butter procedure.

Because we did so much industrial medicine, I had a case referred to me by a GP in the area. A man had become ill working on a bridge nearby. The bridge was being replaced and the old one was to be sold for scrap. This man worked for the company that had won the bid to scrap the old bridge. The contract warned that the bridge had been painted multiple times with lead-based paint, but this apparently didn't mean much to the company. They had sent a crew of iron workers to cut up the old bridge with cutting torches. By the middle of the first day the men were all complaining of feeling sick, but the foreman told them they were just coming down with the flu and to keep working. The patient was the only worker to show up for work the second day and had to quit by noon. Using the cutting torch apparently vaporized the lead, and the men were inhaling it. This patient had the highest serum levels of lead recorded at that time from an inhalation exposure. I hospitalized him and contacted the toxicology department at UC San Francisco. Working with them, I started him on a chelating agent (a substance that will attach itself to a particular atom) by IV, which would bind to the lead and start to remove it from his body. After several days of this, we were able to start him on oral medications and release him from the hospital. Unfortunately, he suffered permanent neural damage and could no longer work as a steel worker because of muscle weakness and loss of coordination. He had no money, and it took years for his lawsuit to come through. The last I heard of him, he had lost his wife but was going to the local junior college learning another trade.

One of the difficulties of a small office is the employees wanting to get their care from "their" doctors. In many respects it's similar to working on your own family and most doctors try to avoid it. One night I got a call from one of our medical assistants saying she had gotten depressed and taken nearly a hundred tricyclic antidepressants. She agreed to meet me at the ER and I went right down. The story was that she had been using cocaine and was trying to get off, but the down of withdrawal was so extreme, she had been placed on antidepressants. As I was taking the history and waiting for the ipecac we'd given her to work, she suddenly stopped talking and went unconscious. I immediately placed a tube in her stomach and washed out as much of the medication as possible. Her body temperature had dropped quite severely, which is a symptom of tricyclic overdose, and she began to have cardiac rhythm problems. This is usually due to pH problems, and we had to get the temperature under control as well as correct her pH. We put her in the ICU, and I spent the entire night following her temps and blood pH and correcting as necessary. By morning, she seemed to stabilize, and I was able to get some sleep. She finally woke up, and we were able to discharge her in a few days and arrange for her to see a psychiatrist. She eventually returned to work but continued to battle the cocaine probably until she left us.

We had hired a new medical assistant, and she asked if I would look at her husband. He was in his early thirties and coached Little League. He always had the kids run one lap of the field to warm up, and he would run with them. He was finding he could no longer keep up, and he had also developed a cough. We had recently expanded our building and added x-ray and mammograms to our available testing. I examined the man and found his breath sounds were unlike anything I'd heard before, so I ordered a chest x-ray.

I made a mistake because both the patient and his wife were standing behind me when I pulled the film from the developer and put it on the screen. His entire right chest was filled with a large mass with about one inch of lung tissue around it. He immediately had questions, and I had to explain there certainly were problems but I didn't know what they were yet. The differential for this huge mass would be either lymphoma or sarcoidosis. Sarcoid is a strange disease, which most commonly occurs in blacks from the South. In spite of that, anyone can turn up with it, and fortunately he proved positive when we got a needle biopsy. He responded very well to the steroids used for this disorder and was back running with the kids in a few months.

Bookkeepers are frequently a problem in a medical office. When we started the group, we hired a bookkeeper who had been working for our Ob-Gyn, but she had more responsibility than she'd ever coped with in her life. Things came to a head when she forgot to send the payroll withholding to the IRS. We caught the error and made an agreement with them that if we had to borrow the money to get it in right away, they wouldn't charge interest and penalties. We did, and the next thing we knew we received a bill for interest and penalties. When we called the IRS, a new person answered and said he wasn't bound by the previous man's agreement. We were out about $7,000 and the bookkeeper quit.

The next bookkeeper was a lady who had worked for a CPA in another state. She seemed quite competent, and our CPA checked her out and agreed. She did quite well for a couple years, but then one of my partners got called to the ER to see her. She was very drunk and had been cut up by her boyfriend. He got her sewed up and watched her overnight. We told her we couldn't have that sort of thing, and if there were any more alcohol problems, she would be fired. The police had filed some charges against her, and she had to hire a lawyer, which she told us was very expensive.

A month or so later I was checking the books in the office on a weekend when I was on call when I found there were two paychecks to the bookkeeper in one pay period. I looked back and found the same pattern in the previous pay period. Checks required the signature of two of the four physician owners, and she had carefully taken one to one pair of docs and the second to the other two so no-one noticed the second paycheck. I called our accountant, and he agreed to be there first thing Monday morning and do a spot audit and confront her with the evidence. He did so, and we learned she was giving the second check to her lawyer to get him paid. We ended up having to fire her and having to explain to the employees who thought she was just injured and lost some time. Many, if not most, physicians have had problems with embezzlement at one time or other, I knew one physician who told me his bookkeeper made more one year than he did. I'm sorry to say he did not prosecute and didn't even put it into her recommendations because he felt stupid. The last he heard of her she was working at the same job in another office in another town.

I had one patient come in with a severe back spasm with which he was barely able to walk. He was a carver and had a show the next day in a town about three hundred miles away. On exam he had nerve involvement and likely a disc extrusion (we didn't have MRI yet), so I told him we'd have to hospitalize him to control the pain and spasm. He refused and said he had to go to his show. I gave him what I could as an outpatient and helped him out to his car in our lot. It turned out to be a very low-slung sports car, so I told his wife, who was driving, that when they got home and she couldn't get him out of the car she should just drive to the ER and honk her horn. I went over to the ER, and sure enough, they showed up a little while later and with the help of two male aids and myself we got him out of the car and onto the gurney. He was in the hospital three days before we got his pain under control.

I had my own personal medical emergency about this time. I had a strep throat probably caught from one of the children in the practice and was on a course of antibiotics. I was leaving the office for the hospital at noon when I realized I didn't have my medication. I went to our sample closet and got another antibiotic, which would kill strep and took that. When I was about halfway to the hospital, my scalp began to itch. By the time I got to the hospital I was having trouble judging oncoming traffic to make the left turn into the ER. Since I was the chief of the ER committee, the ER doc seemed to be hesitant to treat me. The chief ER nurse called our office for help, and they told him I was in the hospital. He responded that he *knew* that and asked for my partner. My blood pressure was 50/0 and they were giving me doses of adrenaline when I heard the ER nurse comment on all the heart arrhythmias they were causing. I was also given large doses of antihistamine, and when my partner got there, they went to steroids, which finally got things under control. Then we realized I had just taken the medication, and it probably wasn't totally absorbed so they gave me medication to make me vomit up any remaining drug. I threw up so hard the blood vessels in my eyes ruptured. I was never sure whether the anaphylaxis or the treatment was worse.

After a number of years I was elected the president of the county medical society. One of the things on my agenda was to develop a speaker's bureau to talk about the costs of medical care, which had been rising rapidly for a number of years. This issue is still relevant today and though the causes have never changed, the politicians have never figured it out. There are three causes underlying these increases. First, technology is constantly advancing, resulting in much improved testing and treatment options, but each new option seems to be more expensive than the last. We've gone from x-rays to CT scans to MRIs to PET scans for example, each one costing a multiple of the last. Second, our population is ageing and therefore using more and more medical care. Over half of your lifetime medical expenses are spent in the last six months of life. And finally, there is the general underlying rate of inflation, which affects everything. What does not underlie these increased costs is fraud and abuse, which the politicians always claim they can correct to control expenses. There is no question there is fraud and abuse in the system, but that is not the major cause of the higher cost of medicine. We won't be able to control costs without rationing and generally that is unacceptable to the American people.

Our medical society represented two counties because the county just north of us was too small to have its own. That isolation seemed to draw physicians who didn't want scrutiny, and since I was the president of the society, we had to deal with the complaints. The investigator for the state licensing bureau would stop as a courtesy and tell me what he was looking into on each visit. He also wanted to know if I had any complaints that might end up in his lap. He told me one time his work load would be greatly reduced if he wasn't responsible for that other county.

One time a candidate for president of the state medical society came up to speak, and we were discussing our speaker's bureau when I mentioned we didn't try to defend physicians who were making $500,000 or more as some were. He gave me a funny look and I realized he was one of them. He was rather cold the rest of the evening. Probably a good thing I wasn't looking to run for state office.

One day I was in the next town helping the local hand surgeon on a tendon release when the nurse came running in and told me they needed me in the next OR. They had had a young man brought in with a self-inflicted shotgun wound to the abdomen, and he was bleeding hard. They had found one of the general surgeons making rounds and pulled him into the OR as well. I was a little concerned because this guy was fine outside the OR but had a reputation as a screamer when things got tense. Anesthesia had two large bore IVs going with blood pumps and was still slowly losing ground. We rapidly opened the abdomen and found the left lobe of the liver as well as the small bowel and the large bowel had all been hit. The bleeding was coming from the liver. My job was primarily to suction the blood so the surgeon could see what he was doing. My one suction was insufficient, and they ended up running a suction line across the hall from a vacant OR. With these I was barely able to keep up with the bleeding. The surgeon turned the cautery machine on high and was finally able to seal off most of the bleeding. We fixed the holes in the large bowel and flushed out the abdomen and were able to close with our patient still alive. I was amazed that there had been no screaming probably because he was concentrating so hard. I ran into the surgeon a few weeks later, and he told me that after seven more surgeries and one trip to the psych ward, the patient had left the hospital in good shape at least physically.

It was impossible to avoid the legal profession, and they often were looking for someone to review malpractice cases. My first involvement occurred when an attorney from Los Angeles named me in a suit against my residency program because my name was on the chart. I had seen the patient both before and after the incident but was home asleep when the problem occurred. I was senior resident on both OB and Surgery at the time, and when my junior resident called to say he was having a problem, I had been up for twenty-four hours straight. I told him to get the attending in because I didn't feel I was safe to be dealing with complications. He called the junior attending, and they handled the problem using a rather old method. The lawyer let me know that if I would testify against them, he would remove my name from the suit. I told him since I wasn't there and had never used the technique in question I could not form an opinion. He dropped my name anyway.

I was hired to be a defense witness in a malpractice action against an FP in the southern part of our county. The case involved a lady who came to the hospital in early labor and began to pass blood. The physician came from home and immediately recognized she had a placenta previa (placenta across the opening of the uterus). He called the city near us to arrange transfer because he didn't have the facilities to do a Cesarean. He got two units of blood on the ambulance and got her on her way in about twenty minutes. The patient arrived at the larger hospital and was taken immediately to the OR where a C-section was done. The baby came out very depressed and underwent what I thought was a not-very-aggressive resuscitation. The outcome was that the baby ended up with permanent neurological damage. I reviewed the chart first and felt the doc had done everything he could and amazingly fast. He was working with a twenty-bed hospital with two nurses on the night shift and immediately recognized what was happening. Subsequently I was deposed by the plaintiff's lawyer. This guy came from Los Angeles and his expert was an Ob-Gyn who had never worked in a rural area or in a small hospital. The lawyer kept asking the same questions over and over in an effort to get me to change my testimony. Since I was being paid $400 an hour, I was perfectly happy to keep repeating my answer. Shortly after this, I was informed that the case had been dropped, and I like to hope it was due to my testimony. I thought there was a good case against the pediatrician but nobody asked.

The very obese patient who had had the placenta previa earlier returned pregnant again and even heavier than ever. I talked with her about weight and diet throughout her pregnancy, but it had no effect. In fact, one of my other patients told me that she would brag about ignoring my instructions. I even put a note in her chart after one session, saying I had told her that if she didn't stop gaining, it was possible that either she or her baby could die. When she came to term, she weighed 280 pounds and was 4 feet 10 inches. We had her scheduled for a repeat C-section, and she was admitted at about thirty-nine weeks gestation (forty is term) for her repeat surgery. The anesthesiologist felt she was way too heavy for a spinal to be placed and set her up for a "crash" induction. In those circumstances we had to have the baby out by about three to five minutes to avoid the anesthetic getting to the infant. At surgery I was assisted by our new Ob-Gyn, and as soon as anesthesia gave us the word, we started. Within two minutes I noticed the blood was very dark, indicating poor oxygenation, and I asked the anesthesiologist what was wrong, and he told me he couldn't intubate her and was unable to get sufficient oxygen by mask. I told my assistant we had to hurry and get the baby out, which we did. Without the baby and amnionic fluid under her diaphragms, anesthesia was able to bag her with a mask and the color of the blood improved. The nurse anesthetist came in during the procedure and tried to intubate her as he was the one who had done so with her first child, but he too was unable to get a good airway. The ENT surgeon also tried with a different instrument but was unable to get the tube in, and he left. When we finished the surgery, I asked the anesthesiologist how things were going and he told me he was able to keep going with a mask but he had not used any anesthetic other than the initial IV induction drugs throughout the procedure. I immediately recognized she was in extremely serious trouble and practically forced the ENT to come in and do a tracheotomy to get a better airway. Just as we finished this procedure, the patient arrested, and we were unable to get her back. I was in a daze when I had to go talk to the husband and tell him his wife died of an anesthesia mishap. He asked me what would happen next, and I told him it would be a coroner's case because all deaths in the OR were looked into by the coroner.

The baby did fine and went home in two or three days with the husband and his mother-in-law who was an ex-nurse from our ER. They were both pretty hostile, and I tried to understand their view. Naturally, a few months later, a suit was filed against me, the anesthesiologist, and the hospital as well as the ENT. The anesthesiologist carried no malpractice insurance and had been hiding his assets for years, so he immediately declared bankruptcy and was subsequently removed from the suit. After the malpractice trial the bankruptcy was disallowed by the courts, but it had served its purpose and he never went on trial.

The trial itself, which occurred several years after the incident, was a nonstop nightmare. The plaintiffs had hired a malpractice firm from the Bay Area, and they sent a young and very arrogant lawyer with little experience who came with a collection of hired gun experts. One of them was a well-known anesthesiologist we calculated had made enough from this case to buy himself a new Mercedes. I couldn't understand why a man with his reputation would lower himself to such an extent, so I called a friend of mine who was an anesthesiologist practicing in the Bay Area, and he told me the man was so nasty the residents in his program had rebelled and he had been demoted from department chair and assigned no further residents. My friend said ever since that had happened, he had been gunning for any physician he could get.

While picking the jury, we had one crazy woman who badly wanted on the panel and claimed to have no contact with our office when in fact her daughter had been a C-section patient of mine and she and her husband were patients of my partners. At the very time she was on the stand, her husband was putting lines in our parking area to work off some of their bills. I told my lawyer about this and he challenged her and got her off the jury pool. She was furious and indeed turned up as a paid witness against me claiming her daughter wasn't warned that she could die with a C-section.

It took over a week just to pick the jury and the whole nightmare lasted six weeks. During opening statements, the plaintiff brought his two boys to court, and my attorney took advantage of that to point to them and state they would not be alive without me. They never were to be seen for the rest of the trial.

The plaintiff's hired guns included the above-mentioned anesthesiologist, who testified the error was inducing anesthesia with a non-reversible muscle relaxant. Once that drug was given, the anesthesiologist was stuck with finding some way to breathe for the patient. Since the anesthesiologist was no longer a defendant, the plaintiff's expert claimed I had erred by not going to the head of the table and taking over even though the anesthesiologist, the anesthetist, and the ENT were all airway specialists and were all there.

The plaintiff's OB specialist was from a Hollywood hospital and admitted to testifying in twenty-six malpractice cases, all for the plaintiffs. He admitted he did three C-sections in the past year (I did at least three per month and our expert averaged three per week).

The hospital's lawyer brought in an expert who did a great deal of research in obesity to explain that the decedent's life expectancy was much decreased by her weight. This information was speaking to the amount of award if we should lose. The plaintiff countered by bringing an elderly physician who testified he'd seen lots of older obese people. My attorney didn't even bother to cross examine him.

I spent two days on the stand and got to explain the feeling I had at the time and continued to hold that all I could do was get the baby out as quickly as possible to save the baby from dying from hypoxia and to relieve the abdominal pressure so it was easier to ventilate the mother. I had to be a little careful because the plaintiff was suing the hospital, claiming they shouldn't have given privileges to the anesthesiologist at all, and we didn't want to get into any fights with their defense.

The jury was out only a short time and came back voting for the defense eleven to one. Since this was a civil case, they did not need to be unanimous. The one juror for the plaintiff said later she thought those little boys deserved some money regardless of who was at fault. As usual, the paper had made a big deal of the lawsuit but buried the results deep inside.

The long-term consequences were more than I realized at the time. Much of the fun went out of practice when you saw each patient as a potential lawsuit. My OB practice dropped off radically and mostly became referrals by the other FPs for C-Sections and difficult deliveries. I also would get a letter cut out of magazine letters threatening my life every so often. I was pretty sure this came from the patient's family, and I just ignored them as much as possible.

We continued to do a fair amount of industrial medicine, and we were contacted by the city where our practice was located to do pre-employment physicals. We agreed until they specified back x-rays, which weren't indicated. We tried to explain to them that it had been shown conclusively that back films didn't predict back trouble but did involve a lot of unnecessary radiation. They had brought in a company who contracted to be sure cities' exams were "defensible." These folks didn't even have a physician on their staff, and we pointed out you could defend nearly anything but the people of the city were adamant so we refused the contract.

The redwood mill had contacted us about a chemical line they wanted to put in. While old growth redwood wouldn't get fungus, the younger trees would, so shipments to the east traveling in a warm, moist rail car would frequently arrive with a black fungus on them, and the shipment would be refused by the buyer. Other mills sprayed their lumber with anti-fungus chemicals, and the redwood people wanted to do the same.

We looked over the plans and checked to be sure none of the chemical would back-siphon into the water supply. The company told us it was a closed system but would be cleaned with water from a garden faucet. The chemical they wanted to use was called Pentachlor and had been around for a long time. Even better, there was a urine test for it, which would allow us to monitor the care the men on the line were exhibiting in their use of protective equipment.

We were asked to check the men who wanted to work this line, and we went out to the mill to do histories and physicals to be sure they were healthy to start with. One history was interesting in that one of the men admitted to drinking a case of beer every Friday and Saturday night. The man was nicknamed "Buddha" for reasons of belly size, but we didn't believe anyone could drink that much in one night. The other workers at the mill told us that he indeed could drink that much, and he owned a small bar where many of them had seen him do it. Naturally all his liver studies were elevated, and we excluded him from the chemical line.

Things got started and we quickly identified one worker who refused to wear his rubber gloves and had a large quantity of Pentachlor in his urine tests. He was promptly removed from the line by the company. At this point the union got involved and wanted a different anti-fungal, which was a Canadian product and fairly new. Its toxicity was known only in rats, and there were no tests for exposure. We weren't happy with the change because of the lack of data, but the company was glad not to pay for those urine screenings.

Soon thereafter one of my partners got a call at about 3:00 a.m. that the water in the washing basins at the plant had turned opalescent. When it was traced back, it was found the people responsible for cleaning the chemical line had just thrown the hose into the chemical pool and forgotten to turn it off, resulting in back siphoning into the plant's water supply. Since we had no way to test for exposure, he sent all sixty men to the hospital to get chemistry panels to see if there was any damage and to establish a baseline against which we could compare potential future damage. The poor night lab technician suddenly had patients coming out his ears. There never did appear to be any damage, but it did show that no matter how careful you think you are, some idiot can mess things up.

We had three workers sent in by their boss for chemical coughs. It seemed his small company had contracted with the people at the local paper mill to replace some steel girders in the mill. First the old girders had to be removed. They had been damaged by constant exposure to fumes from hydrochloric acid used in the process of making paper. To remove the girders they had been cutting them out using a cutting torch. When the metal was heated, the chlorine was released and went into the air. They had breathed it, causing lung irritation. I asked them if they were wearing masks, but they said it was too hot to use them. When I called the local inspector for OSHA, he told me it was the responsibility of the employer to see that the employees wore the proper safety equipment. I passed this information along to the employer and told him I wouldn't file a complaint this time, but he needed to take charge because if I ever saw a similar incident, I would have to file. He agreed and understood, so I was quite surprised when the same men came in with the same problem several weeks later. I filed an OSHA complaint and figured we'd lost that account, but after a few weeks, he came in for something else and told me he'd been fined $9,000, but he understood and would continue to come to us although his men wore masks from then on.

We had a large Portuguese population in our area, mostly from the Azores. Apparently our coastal climate was very similar to that of the islands. Most of the men either ran dairies or were fishermen. The women either were housewives or worked in the fish-packing companies. They had a limited number of names and all the women had Maria somewhere in their names. It was a joke among our medical assistants that if you went to the waiting room and called Maria, half the room would stand up. The men were hard workers and good providers but seemed to feel that was the limit of their requirements. I remember one dairyman in particular who told me he "jumped the fence" occasionally. He passed me on the freeway once with what appeared to be a honky-tonk-type girl in his pickup and honked and waved so I would see what he was up to.

This man had a delightful grown daughter, and he brought in a husband for her from the Azores. The daughter brought her intended straight from the plane to my office. It seemed he had had an abscess on his back and had seen a traditional healer in the Azores before leaving. The healer had opened the abscess (which was good) and then tried to sterilize it with wheat he had heated very hot in a frying pan (which was bad). I was confronted with a second-degree burn in an open abscess and a large area of infection. We cleaned him up and started on antibiotics and he recovered nicely. I was surprised the daughter, who had always seemed very much Americanized, did go ahead and marry the fellow who turned out to be a very nice guy.

I had another arranged marriage in the practice. This was a young woman whose family had come from India. Her father owned one of the local motels and the uncle owned another. Both families came to our office, and she came in one day to tell me her father and mother had arranged a marriage with another Indian fellow who also owned a motel and even had the same last name, although he was unrelated. She was taking a writing class from my wife who was teaching at the local state college and chose to write on the issue of arranged marriage versus our method. She pointed out that they had a much lower rate of divorce and thought it was because, in their traditional family, both the man and the woman had their specific duties in the marriage and therefore weren't competing with each other as happened in American marriages. I was glad she was comfortable with it, because she didn't have much choice. We were invited to the wedding, but I had a woman go into labor and didn't get to go. I was terribly disappointed.

We had another international group we cared for. We had been contacted by the Saudi Arabian Consulate to see if we would care for a number of Saudi students who were going to go the local university. They all were studying psychology, and I asked one of the first ones to come in why this was. He told me they were having a very big problem having gone from desert tribesmen to multimillionaires in a few short years. They were getting training to go back and help people to adapt to these changes.

We were given numbers to add to our bills so the consulate could identify which student the bill was for. It seems they have only about thirteen last names in the country and most of the men are named Mohammed, so it was very confusing who we had seen. They themselves were still pretty traditional, and we'd always had our nurse practitioner see their wives. One day one of them called to say his wife was bleeding vaginally, but our nurse practitioner was off that day so the wife was set up with one of my partners. The husband insisted on staying in the exam room, and my partner was very nervous about doing the necessary exam. Maybe it didn't help when I told him he could do the exam but the husband was going to cut off his hand afterward. He later told me the husband sat with his arms crossed and a scowl on his face the whole time.

All these students were given a Pontiac Firebird on arrival. They came in by way of San Diego, and it being the first time away from their somewhat-repressive society, some of them went wild. I had one young man come in complaining of a discharge. When I went to examine him, I found his shorts were stuffed with paper towels which were nearly soaked with pus. It seems he'd met a lady of the night in San Diego but fortunately hadn't caught one of the more resistant strains of gonorrhea they had there, secondary to all the marines coming back from Vietnam. We were able to treat him with the standard treatment at that time, which was two gigantic syringes of penicillin each of which came with a needle that looked more like a nail than a needle. It was not only curative but also educational.

These young men needed some counselors of their own. Alcohol is not only against Islamic tradition, it is illegal in Saudi Arabia, so these young men had not had much exposure. They took to hanging out at a local night club, and one night two of them got into a fight over a girl.

The loser went outside and set the winner's Fire Bird on fire. Shortly thereafter they were all recalled to Saudi Arabia.

One of the difficult things in practice is when you need medical care for yourself. My partner and his wife whose two children I had delivered decided they wanted no more so he asked me to do a vasectomy. I probably averaged one or more per week, so this was no problem until the medical assistants got wind of it. When he came in for his procedure, they had set everything up so none of them needed to be in the room, but they had also smeared fake blood all over a white apron and borrowed a "de-baller" used in cattle from a local large animal vet, which was prominently displayed on the instrument stand. The whole surgery had been decorated with black balloons. My partner took it well and the procedure went as planned.

Sometimes my patients came a long way for their care. I had one young woman who was living in Iran who came in for obstetrical care. She had grown up locally but had married an Iranian student and moved to Iran with him. When she got pregnant, they looked at the local medical care, and she decided to fly back to the United States for her delivery.

Another lady came from a small village in Alaska. She was native, but her husband was a very tall Caucasian who was the law for his whole area. He shaved his head way before it became popular and looked really tough, which he apparently was. He told me tales of chasing down criminals on snowmobiles and even dog sleds. It was good they had come down because she was small but had a large baby (probably because her husband was so big) and ended up having to have a C-section.

When you live in a rural area, the family doctor will be called upon for all kinds of accidents. We went to our daughter's eighth-grade graduation, which was held in the school's multipurpose room and was to be followed by a dance for the graduates. When the formal ceremonies were completed, the kids had to put the folding chairs away so the dance could start. This was a rare event and they were very excited. They were loading the chairs on some carts when I saw one of Bridget's friends get hit from behind by one of the carts. She screamed and fell down. When I got to her, I could see she had a laceration just above her heel. Her dad and I carried her over to the side where I could do a better exam, and I could see the ends of the Achilles tendon, which had been neatly cut in two. Her dad was telling her they'd have to get her sewn up, and everything would be fine. I had to explain to the girl and her parents what had happened and that she would require surgery to repair the tendon and weeks in a cast and months of therapy. They told me where they wanted to go, and I called ahead to alert the orthopedic surgeon what was coming. This young lady had been a budding athlete and was not going to compete for a long time, if ever, just from putting chairs away.

Sue and I were driving on the freeway when the CB radio I had in my truck started to be full of discussion of a car-versus-motorcycle accident just up the road. When we saw it on the other side of a four lane, I crossed over and parked on the side. There was a van sitting on the side with a large dent squarely in the middle of the front and a young man lying on the pavement with a broken motorcycle helmet and a motorcycle lying nearby. I couldn't believe how many people there were who claimed to be EMTs, both I and II, and one lady who claimed to be a paramedic. They all seemed to have stethoscopes and some had blood pressure cuffs and they all wanted to use them. I identified myself as a physician and went about protecting the young man's neck. His pupils were fixed and dilated, and he was showing signs of progressive neurological damage. When the ambulance arrived, they told me they were required by law to take him to the nearest ER, which was the one at the hospital I used, but we didn't have neurosurgery. I strongly advised them to go the one hospital in the county that had a neurosurgeon because it was obvious to me his only chance was if he had an epidural bleed and could get the pressure relieved fast enough. We were within a few hundred yards of the boundary, but they refused to go anywhere but the nearest hospital even though they knew me and knew I was right. I talked to the doc at our ER who told me they put an IV in the young man and shipped him to the hospital I had recommended. It didn't really matter as his CT scan showed diffuse brain damage, and he just went ahead and died.

We frequently entered the hospital by the door by the ER, and as I was coming in to make noon rounds, the ER doc stopped me and asked if I could give him a hand. He'd just had an ambulance in with a mother and two boys. Since the mother seemed injured severely, he wanted to know if I could check out the kids. As I went in, I immediately recognized the wife of a local physician lying unconscious on one gurney, and I found his two kids in the next room. Fortunately the kids knew me, and I was able to calm them down and check them out. They were fine. It was possible to smell alcohol on the mother, and when the husband arrived, he was so angry I thought he might do something to her. I got him to go to the kids and stay out of the way. He admitted to me she had a drinking problem, which they had been trying to deal with but hadn't been successful. The scans showed she had a small contusion directly in the area of the alerting system in the brain. She remained unconscious for several weeks and finally was transferred to a rehab hospital where she slowly woke up but had developed pretty severe contractures of her arms and legs, and when she returned, she required a wheelchair. Shortly after she returned, he divorced her and kept custody of the kids.

We seldom saw dentists at the hospital, but one time the dentist involved must have broken speed records getting there. I was called about a patient who had been in a single car accident where his car left the highway and crashed into a stack of lumber at a lumberyard near the highway. He had moderately severe injuries including several broken teeth. I admitted him to the ICU for observation and asked about his dentist. He told me he'd been having a root canal that morning and had just left the dental office when he apparently passed out. I called his dentist and told him about the broken teeth, and he was in the ICU doing temporaries practically before I hung up. I suspect he was somewhat concerned about malpractice after allowing a patient to drive right after such a procedure.

As time was passing, I found I really enjoyed working in the ER. Working in the ER was both more exciting and paid a little more money. I cut my practice to three days a week and added ER shifts to my schedule.

The ER Years

With my OB practice decreased because of the lawsuit and my reluctance to keep getting up in the night, I also noticed my practice was aging and I was seeing more high blood pressure and diseases of aging. I cut back my practice and started working one day a week in the hospital ER. This didn't pay very well but was often fairly slow, so we worked twenty-four-hour shifts and usually could get some sleep. We had two trauma beds and three other beds. In addition we had radio control of the ambulances and a home alert system for the elderly. That system was frequently a nuisance since if the person didn't reset their device every twenty-four hours, it would alarm, and we would have to call them and get them to hit the reset button. Many of them didn't understand what was needed, and the nurses would end up screaming into the phone at some deaf, elderly patient, trying to explain which button they needed to push. If they didn't answer, we had a list of relatives or friends who would go and check on them, and as a last resort, the police would do a welfare check for us.

Since you were the only doc in the hospital at night, sometimes you'd get called to deal with an urgent problem such as a delivery or a patient out of control. One night I was called to the general nursing floor for an elderly patient who was "sun-downing." This refers to the tendency of some elderly patients to become disoriented when it gets dark outside. This man had broken out a window in his room and was trying to climb out. The nurses were afraid of him because he was sailing pieces of window glass at them like Frisbees. When I got there, he was continuing to refuse to get back in bed and was threatening anyone who came into the room with pieces of glass. I decided there was nothing that could be done but to physically control him and told the nurses to get out the soft restraints. Once they were ready, I went into the room and managed to duck the piece of glass he threw. I grabbed him in a bear hug, pinning his arms to his sides, and since he was pretty frail, I simply picked him up and laid him on the bed where the nurses were able to secure his restraints. I went around in the morning to see how he was doing, and it happened his docs were making rounds. When he saw me, he pointed and said, "Don't mess with that guy. He's tough."

The ER always has its regulars most of whom are addicts trying to get drugs, but some of whom have very real and chronic problems. One fellow we became very familiar with would call the ambulance for various imagined problems. On one occasion he came in claiming he couldn't walk and would have to be admitted. When I went over him, there was no evidence that his legs wouldn't move and really no evidence he was sick in any way except mentally. When I told him he was going to be all right, he refused to leave, claiming his legs wouldn't work. After trying repeatedly to get him to leave, I finally called the police because we needed the space. An officer came in, and I explained to him what was going on. Sure enough, they were familiar with this man as well. The officer went to the bed and engaged the man in conversation. After a little bit he asked if the patient knew what a come-along hold was. When the man said no, the officer said, "Let me show you," which he did, forcing the man out of the gurney and onto his feet. Indeed the patient demonstrated he not only could walk but could do so on his tiptoes.

I had always been suspicious this man might well be dangerous, and indeed there were rumors he beat his parents to prevent them from complaining about him. The next time he came in with another imaginary ailment, I spent some time talking with him, and he finally admitted he really was a CIA agent. If people crossed him, he would have to kill them. That was what we needed to place a 5150 hold for psychiatric evaluation on him, which I signed as did both my ER nurses who heard what he had said. We arranged for transfer to the county psychiatric facility where they had seventy-two hours to evaluate whether he was a danger to himself or others and whether he was able to care for himself. I got a call from a doc who worked at the psych unit doing physicals for new admits. I knew this man because we had fired him from our ER. He never had any training beyond internship and earned most of his living as a carpenter. He told me he didn't see anything wrong with the man and was going to release him. I told him he wasn't a psychiatric specialist and the 5150 was signed by three emergency healthcare professionals, so if he released the man, I would hold him responsible for anything he did. I would also see to it he never practiced medicine in any form ever again. He angrily agreed not to set the man free. When the professional mental health experts got done with him, it turned out he was beating his parents and was also stalking a female ambulance attendant. He'd been sitting outside the call station watching her and sending her letters on stationary he'd stolen from the library using letters he'd cut out of magazines. After the seventy-two-hour hold he was transferred to the state hospital for the criminally insane.

I had finished my shift one night and had changed to my jeans and a sweatshirt to go home. As I was leaving, I was passed by a man carrying a briefcase, and I could see the butt of a gun sticking out of the briefcase. There was an ambulance in, and since the paramedics knew most of the cops including the undercovers, I asked them to look at the sign-in window and see if they knew who this guy was. They said they didn't think he was a cop, so I called 911 and told the police we had a man in the ER with a gun. He had asked for a specific ENT surgeon, and we were very concerned what his intentions were. The nurses moved him to the radiology waiting room, which was empty, and told him there would be a short wait before the requested physician came in. The police arrived and I showed them where he was. They walked in and introduced themselves and took his hand as if to shake it. The next thing the man knew he was in a submission hold and being handcuffed. They found he not only had a loaded .38 in this briefcase, he had a Derringer hidden behind his belt buckle, also loaded. He turned out to be a local defense lawyer; some of his clients had been paying him with cocaine. He'd sniffed so much of this, his nasal septum was ulcerating, and it hurt, which was why he wanted to see the ENT. The police had arrested him for carrying a concealed weapon without a permit. They told me later they'd been called to his house because he'd sniffed so much cocaine, he'd gone off the deep end and started shooting up his house. As a result he was committed to the psychiatric hospital as a danger to himself and others.

I've read that the national average is one violent episode per ER per day. Our little ERs didn't reach that level, but we had quite a few. One occurred when I wasn't working and was very glad not to have participated. A man entered the ER with a pistol and demanded drugs. Naturally, he was given everything he wanted. As he was leaving, he fired his gun to emphasize they weren't to follow him. He shot into the solid core door on the entrance, and the bullet penetrated the door and hit a white coat hanging on the back of the door, and it fell to the floor. A nurse's aide was standing just behind the door, and he told me later he nearly fainted. Our hospital was on the edge of town and had empty fields surrounding it. This guy took off across the field on foot, and by the time he got across, the cops were waiting there to meet him. The cops told me later they knew him very well because his brother had just been convicted of an axe murder. Nice family.

Our hospital was backed up against a field, which ended at the freeway. There was a freeway exit about half a mile from us. One evening I got a call from the ambulance giving us a heads-up that they had been called for a single-car rollover accident near our exit, so they would be getting to us faster than normal. We went ahead and cleared out our trauma beds and waited. The radio came to life with the statement that there were "kids all over the freeway." Naturally we had contingency plans for mass causalities, and although these weren't mass causalities, they were probably going to be more than I could handle alone. I called a code "Orange," which got me a couple extra nurses from elsewhere in the hospital and meant I had to call the other two ERs in the area and arrange for them to help. My paramedics had called for a backup ambulance and had begun triaging the victims. There were seven children and three adults of whom two were alive. The third adult was pronounced on scene. To make things worse, they were Hmong and spoke very little English. We had a colony of Hmong in the area after a local church sponsored some Hmong families after Vietnam, and several others had joined the original group.

I had agreed with the other ERs that I would take the two worst-injured kids and the worst adult, and they would handle the lesser injuries and walking wounded. When my patients arrived, the "worst" of the kids was dead, and we were unable to resuscitate as is so common in kids and trauma. We were able to stabilize the other child and the adult, and they both went to surgery for orthopedic injuries and were placed on head trauma watch. I think the paramedics simply didn't have the heart to pronounce the child on scene and I couldn't blame them.

One morning I was driving into the hospital to start my eight o'clock shift when I noticed some black smoke along the freeway. The location was one of those trailer parks where the trailers are either single wide or travel trailers and pretty sleazy. When I got to the ER, I learned there had been one person injured in a trailer fire who would be arriving soon.

The injured, when it arrived, was a woman with severely burned hands. The story was that the family lived in one of the travel trailers and had no heat. She had taken the baby with her while she walked the five-year-old to the bus stop for his kindergarten bus. She had left the oven on to heat the trailer because it was a cold morning. When she got back, she found her trailer fully involved in flames with her two- and four-year-olds trapped inside. She had tried to get them out but couldn't go in the door, so she'd tried to pull off the aluminum off the side of the trailer severely burning her hands. She was, of course, completely hysterical and in severe pain. We got IVs in her and started pain medications. I was ordering dressings when I looked around and found I didn't have any nurses. I found them in the office crying, and I had to be very firm to get them to go back to work. I pointed out I wasn't feeling so well myself, but she was our first priority. One of the things I had to watch was the tendency to tell her it would be OK because it wouldn't be OK. We got her stabilized and arranged transfer to a hand plastics surgeon with extensive experience with hand burns. As we were finishing up, her husband arrived, and I was impressed that after I told him what had happened he went right to her and held her, rather than worrying about his own feelings. Child deaths are always the most difficult for ER personnel to deal with.

After I'd been working at our ER for a short period of time, I was contacted by an ER group in San Francisco who contracted with small rural hospitals to provide ER coverage.

They had a small hospital about sixty miles from us where they needed more docs to work in the ER. Although the hospital was small, the ER saw about twenty-five thousand patients a year because the town was very short of physicians. The ER docs worked twelve-hour shifts and were paid very well. We had a physician's assistant who came in about 10:00 a.m. and worked twelve hours. The rest of the time we were alone, and like my hospital, there were frequently no other docs in the building at night. They did have a CT scanner but only one radiologist who wouldn't let us use it unless she was there. If she decided it was her night off we had x-ray only. There was also only one general surgeon and one orthopedic surgeon, so back-up was sketchy.

The town itself was very isolated and none of the ER docs lived there. The ER group bought a house and hired maid service so ER docs had a place to stay between shifts. The only industries were a new large prison, fishing, and some tourism. The tourism consisted mostly of retirees who had RVs and stayed on the beach in an area where they were allowed to park for free. Many of them would surf fish, but others were just there to avoid the heat of summer by being on the cool ocean. These folks were always a problem because they had no medical records and were not particularly sophisticated when it came to giving medical history. They would come in requesting refills on their yellow pills and not even be sure what these pills were for.

Soon after I started there, we began so see men with steel foreign bodies in their corneas. It seemed the new prison had had its locks improperly installed, and the guards had noticed prisoners wandering around when they were supposed to be locked up. These men with the foreign bodies worked for a security lock company in New York and were staying there to fix the locks. They had to remove the old locks, which were riveted into place, so there was nothing a prisoner could unscrew. This meant grinding each rivet off before the lock could be replaced. They frequently would get tiny particles of steel in their eyes, and they would then come to the ER to get these removed.

One of the problems with working with steel was that in the salty tears of the eye they would rust and form a "rust ring" around the particle, which would affect vision. If they came in quickly enough, the ring would be small, but if they waited even a few hours, it could become a major problem. Fortunately the hospital had invested in a slit lamp, which is an instrument used to see the eye well, and using this device, we were usually able to remove the metal particle and "polish" (use a burr to cut) out the rusty cornea surface so it could heal without the ring. This is always a little scary since you absolutely don't want to perforate the cornea, but with lots of practice it became routine.

The prison was an interesting place in that no one went there for what they'd done before they got into the prison system. Most of these guys had tried to kill a guard or another prisoner. When one of my friends who was a local cop was taken on a tour of the prison, he noticed they had both bars and inch-thick glass. When he asked why they needed both, the guards said they'd tried just bars but the prisoners kept throwing feces and urine on them through the bars, so the glass was added.

Since the prison was a major employer in the area, we saw quite a few of the guards in the ER. I often felt there was little difference between some of the guards and the prisoners. One guard came in with a swollen hand after a fight in a bar. He had a "boxer's fracture" of the fifth metacarpal on his right hand. He was very upset because he was afraid he wouldn't be able to do his job with a splint or cast in place. I asked what his job involved, and he said he was a "shooter." This meant he stood watch in a tower with an AR 15 automatic rifle, and if a prisoner crossed a line near the fence, his job was to shoot. His problem was his weapon was military style and therefore didn't have a bolt with a handle but rather had a straight piece of metal sticking out and the weapon was cocked by hitting that with the side of the hand right where his fracture was. I went ahead and put him into a very heavy splint made of fiberglass and told him to see the orthopedic surgeon in a few days and had to hope I had reinforced it enough to allow him to be able to cock his weapon. He was afraid his boss would fire him for getting into a fight anyway.

The prison had its own infirmary and three docs who were employed by the state, but none of them spoke English very well. None of them wanted anything to do with any significant disease or injury so they sent a lot of prisoners down to the local ERs.

The prisoners from the penitentiary were such consummate liars they could look you in the eye and nearly convince you of something even when you knew they were lying. One such prisoner was brought in because he had begun having “convulsions” for no apparent reason. Naturally I was suspicious, and when he had a “convulsion” in the ER, I decided to test him and in the midst of his “convulsion,” I put a cotton bud directly against his cornea and he showed no response. Since he didn’t blink I admitted him over night until an EEG (brain wave test) could be done the next morning. The next time I worked, I checked on him and found he had a normal EEG and had been sent back to the prison.

One evening we got a radio call from the ambulance that they had been called to the prison, and they were doing a trauma code. Trauma codes seldom work, but this one did get the man restarted. The story was that he’d been lifting weights (one of the few recreational activities they were allowed). When he was bench pressing 250 pounds, two of his fellow prisoners pushed down on the bar, which fell and finally stopped about three-quarters of an inch into his forehead. We had no neurosurgeons, so I called the airport and had them get the fixed wing medevac plane ready to transport him the 135 miles over the mountains to the closest neurosurgical facility. When he arrived at the ER, he was completely out of his head and swinging at anyone who came close. We managed to pin his arm and get an IV in it and injected him with a paralyzing agent. We then intubated him and got him thoroughly restrained as well. Since he would have to be in the air a while, I sent a nurse with him with an additional vial of the medicine in case the first wore off before arrival. She also would bag him all the way since he was paralyzed. When the ambulance left the ER, we noted he’d only been in the ER for about thirty minutes and he arrived at the neurosurgeons in good shape considering. I saw in the paper that he’d gone to surgery and was doing well. I had to wonder if I had done society any favors by saving a man who was convicted of first-degree murder, second-degree murder, and armed robbery, but it wasn’t my job to judge.

I was actually working in my hospital’s ER when the guards brought a prisoner in from sixty miles away. These were such bad guys they normally sent four guards with them when they had to transport them, but this guy had six guards. He'd been stabbed in the neck with what they call an ice pick, which is any thin, pointed weapon. This had been made out of a piece of oven grill with one end sharpened and the other covered with tape to make a crude handle. It had entered his neck about a millimeter anterior to the carotid artery and was pushed in with such force it had stuck in the front of one of the cervical vertebrae. The man was lying on the gurney being absolutely still. When I went to examine him, the head guard handed his gun to one of the other guards who put his back to the wall with the gun pointing to the ceiling, and the head guard came and stood right beside me. After I'd called the ENT surgeon to come in and take care of this problem, I asked the guard why so much extra security. He told me this was one of the most dangerous prisoners they had. It seemed this little 5'5" Mexican was the enforcer for one of the prison gangs, and all that happened was another gang's enforcer got to him first. It was pretty obvious the attacker knew what he was aiming for; he'd simple missed. I was later told by the ENT that one of the guards had even come into the OR and stood against the wall with a gun while the prisoner was under anesthesia.

The PAs working in the smaller hospital's ER were very different. One was very experienced and had excellent judgment. The second one was trained in the military and was weak in the judgment department so I had to keep closer track of what he was doing. The more experienced one was pretty much able to work on his own and only occasionally needed input from me, but the other one had to be watched. On a very busy day I was working with him when I saw the nurse bringing in a pediatric lumbar puncture tray. Since I hadn't ordered it, I asked what it was for. She said the PA had asked for it. This is not a procedure I would let a PA do unless I knew he was very competent with it. I asked the PA to come back to the office and asked him why he wanted to do an LP on an infant. He said he had an eighteen-month-old with a fever of 104.6 and was worried about meningitis. I asked about any signs of meningitis such as stiff neck, and he admitted there were no such signs. I suggested he have the nurses get the temp down and then see if there was anything other than the ear infection he had already identified. After fever-controlling measures were implemented, there was no evidence of any meningeal irritation. He apparently was totally unaware that high fever was fairly typical of pediatric ear infections.

After 10:00 p.m. the PA went home and the doc was on his own. Fortunately most nights the night ER nurse was a lady who had been the head nurse in a major city ER and was probably as, if not more, knowledgeable than my PAs. One night we had a man come in who was complaining of severe abdominal pain, and just as I finished examining him, he threw up at least two units of blood. I got a large bore IV in one arm while she got another in the other arm, and we started pouring fluids in while I passed a nasogastric tube, which showed very little blood left in the stomach. We put the tube to suction and got the lab busy setting up blood and transferred him to the ICU to be cared for by one of the staff internists. We both just looked at our ER, which had blood all over. Finally the only thing we could do with the gurney was to wheel it outside and flush it down on the grass. As far as I know grass won't get AIDS or hepatitis B. I suspect that technique is not in the OSHA handbook.

Sometimes OSHA has unrealistic expectations in their regulations, probably because the regulations are written by bureaucrats rather than physicians or nurses. When I started the IV in the patient who was vomiting blood, he was in shock and had very little blood pressure which made his veins very hard to feel. I was just getting the IV in place when the head nurse of the hospital walked in and became very upset because I wasn't wearing gloves. She said there was a $6,000 fine if OSHA caught me starting an IV without gloves. I pointed out I'd started out with gloves but couldn't feel the vein with such low pressure. I felt it was better to keep the man alive even if we did get fined than to let him die in order to follow a regulation. After years of practice I've gotten pretty good at hitting veins with gloves on, but sometimes I need to identify the vein first with my bare finger.

In my old hospital's ER the head nurse was a male nurse who was sometimes a bit of a practical joker. One day he brought a patient back to see me who claimed to be the patient of a doc who was out of town. He claimed to have had a car transmission fall on his forearm, and he just wanted some pain meds. He was wearing long sleeves and his hand and lower forearm had no bruising. Alarm bells were going off in my head so I looked at his arm and then pushed up his sleeve to where I could see the needle tracks in the anticubital fossa (front of the elbow). I suggested he didn't have a crush injury but rather a vein problem. I looked up to see the ER nurse grinning from ear to ear. I said, "You knew him, didn't you?" He agreed he did, and I asked him why he hadn't warned me and he said he knew the guy wouldn't get past me, but he wanted to see how long it took me to catch him.

I was working the old ER when a family brought in an elderly relative with severe abdominal pain. He was in his early nineties and was severely distended. They told me this had been going on for three days and seemed to be getting worse. His abdomen was "tympanitic" (sounded like a drum when thumped). X-ray showed much of his bowel had air-fluid levels, indicating it wasn't working. All this added up to a terrible syndrome caused by a clot in the mesenteric artery. The only treatment is to remove most of the small bowel and to reconnect what one surgeon called his appetite to his a—hole. The patient had a private physician, and while we waited for him to arrive, I explained to the family what was going on and that there was very little hope. I told them that if he was my relative, I would admit him for pain control and expect he would die in a day or two. The private physician was known to me to be very interested in money, and when he arrived he called a surgeon with similar views and they convinced the family that what was really needed was immediate surgery. His physician tried to put an endotracheal tube in place and was doing such a butcher job, I took the instrument away from him and did it myself. They rushed off to surgery and the poor old man died in the ICU the next day, but they had charged Medicare about an additional $10,000+ in the meantime. I lost a lot of respect for those two physicians.

I happened to be working in my hospital's ER when a large quake hit in the San Francisco area resulting in collapsed freeways and fires from broken gas lines. At first the reports were very sketchy, and I began to wonder what would happen if most of the ERs in the Bay Area were closed down and how far they would be sending injured. As it happened, the ERs had only minor damage and were functional, but it did raise a strong question about what would happen if the "big one" struck.

Since I was working two ERs and had been in the military I was asked to be the chairman of our hospital's disaster-planning committee. I've always found disaster planning to be very interesting. We wrote up a general disaster plan with various contingencies and then had to test the plan to see where the shortcomings were since you usually don't get it completely right the first time. We held a drill with a bunch of high school students who volunteered to play the victims. The scenario was a bus accident, and we made up the students in my group's parking lot. The other hospitals in the area participated by counting beds and letting us know how many injuries they each could take. Our hospital actually cleared and moved beds around and found the necessary surgeons and OR crews. The paramedics were expected to triage the patients (decide who went first), and the students were transported to the hospital with the worst injuries first and only after these were under control, did they simulate taking others to the other hospitals. All in all it went pretty well, and after a big meeting of everyone involved, we agreed to do another in a year.

The following year we did a simulated air plane crash, and one of the airlines even let us borrow an aircraft for a few hours. I discovered we actually had a complete military field hospital at our airport, but we didn't break it out for a small exercise. Things were going well until the fire chief called to say they had detected radiation on the plane. I had no idea what the levels he reported meant but was very upset the information came so late that we had contaminated all three ERs in the exercise. Most of what the plane would carry would be diagnostic isotopes for our scanners, and indeed when I talked to the radiologist, the amount of contamination was so small it would have caused no major problems. As a result of these drills, I was asked to take the job of county airport disaster coordinator, which basically meant keeping track of our surplus MASH hospital.

When I worked in the small hospital ER, we frequently had contact with the Native American population. These patients had a big problem with alcohol, and their visits were frequently alcohol related. One afternoon I had a call from the ambulance that they had been called to a truck-versus-tree accident. There were three teenage Native American males involved, and the fire department was coding one of them. When they arrived in the ER, it only took a few seconds to see that the coded young man was dead and wasn't going to be revived. One of the young men had minor injuries and the third was screaming about back pain. We shot a cross table x-ray and discovered he essentially had no L-4 vertebra. This vertebra was "exploded" and fragments had gone in all directions. The fire department and the paramedics had done a wonderful job in getting him to the hospital neurologically intact. We got him stabilized and I called the nearest neurosurgeon about transfer, but he didn't have the necessary rods to stabilize the back and really didn't want the case anyway. We called the next nearest hospital with neurosurgical facilities, and they said they could take him and did have the necessary internal fixation devices. We flew him there, and the last I heard he was doing well post op and had full use of his legs.

While we were busy with the young man with the exploded vertebra, one of the volunteer firemen approached me and asked if I could draw blood on the patient who had expired. When I looked up, it was apparent this man had been giving this young man mouth to mouth during the code at the scene, and he had blood all around his mouth. I really had no idea what the legal implications were, but after asking the highway patrol officer there, I went ahead and obtained blood for a HIV test as well as Hepatitis B. I had never tried to draw blood from a corpse but it went fine, and I felt this fireman deserved the reassurance a negative test would confer. Today with modern drugs we might have placed the fireman on HIV drugs until the test was completed.

Another alcohol problem I encountered at this hospital started one morning when the ambulance called to tell us they were going to a local motel to pick up two unconscious men. These were two well-known Native American alcoholics who would panhandle around town. They were brothers, and apparently had gotten hold of more money than usual. They had bought a bottle of whisky and rented the motel room. They apparently had drunk the whisky like they normally would wine. When they arrived in the ER, they had the highest blood alcohol I had ever seen. Blood alcohols of 0.08 are the legal limit for driving and these fellows were both above 0.6. I was unaware this level was ever compatible with life. One of the brothers had very serious changes in his liver enzymes, and I admitted him to the ICU. The other seemed to be tolerating things fairly well so I put him in our holding room, which had a glass window just behind our desk, and had monitors, which had repeaters on our desk. We put an IV in him and ran in a fructose solution, which is supposed to help. Over several hours he began waking up although his blood alcohol was still high enough that a normal person should have been unconscious. He decided he needed to go to the bathroom and started to climb out of bed. My nurse ran in to stop him, but he managed to climb out over the raised sides and was starting to shuffle along looking for the bathroom. With each step there was a "plop" behind him. After the nurses got him under control they ended up in a fight with housekeeping as to who had to clean up the mess. Housekeeping won by refusing to even come down and look.

This patient was eventually discharged. Even though his blood alcohol was still high we felt it was probably near his normal. When I came back for my next shift, I found his brother had died a couple days later from severe acute alcoholic hepatitis.

I was driving home after working an all-night shift when I woke up driving on the gravel at the side of the road. and I decided I had to change my lifestyle if I was going to live very long. I began to explore the job openings available. One opening that appealed to me was a job teaching in a Family Practice residency in the mountain states. I called and talked to the director, and he was especially interested in my OB experience and wanted to talk to me about the job of OB director. He did want someone quickly, and I explained we had a malpractice "tail," which was over $49,000. My contract said that if I gave six months' notice the group would pay it but less time would be prorated. He seemed to feel that would be no problem, and if I was hired the hospital where the residency was located would take care of it. He asked me to fly out and interview, so Sue and I made arrangements to do so.

When we got there, we found a town that I thought would be very nice, and the residency director showed us around the hospital. He had asked me to do a lecture for the residents but hadn't told me very much about what, so I had prepared a talk on recognizing term and when to intervene in extended pregnancies. The first day I was asked to lunch by the Ob-Gyn who ran the department, and it didn't take long to recognize he didn't like FPs getting into his rice bowl. It was apparent there were turf wars in this department. When it came time for my lecture, I discovered they all had small ultrasounds in their OB exam rooms and simply got an ultra sound almost every visit and used that to determine gestation. We had never been able to afford such a set up and so had to send the patient to the hospital for an ultrasound, which was read by the radiologist. These residents were quite certain they would have their ultrasounds in their offices, and my information really wasn't relevant to them. I could only open the lecture to questions they might want answered, but all in all, the experience stunk. I then met with the financial officer at the hospital who had no intention of paying for the insurance tail and suggested I could use my buy-out from the group to cover it.

Sue and I discussed all this on the way home and I called back to tell the director I was no longer interested. I really wanted to beat him to the punch because, after that lecture, I wouldn't have hired me and I was sure the residents had felt the same.

I continued to work two ERs and part-time in the office. I was in our hospital's ER when the ambulance called to say they had been dispatched to a police action where there were two victims. They called back a few minutes later to say one of the victims was dead on scene, and they were coding the other. When they arrived, they had an elderly man who was in complete arrest. The story was that he had a schizophrenic son who had had some sort of upset. This young man was an aficionado of martial arts, and when he became upset he'd started chasing his father and brought him down with a throwing knife in the back. The mother had locked herself in the house and called 911. When the sheriff arrived, the young man hurled a throwing star at the deputy who told him to stop. Rather than stopping, he threw another, which the deputy ducked and at the same time put three bullets in the young man's chest. When the ambulance arrived, they found the old man lying in a large pool of blood with the knife lying near him. He apparently was still barely alive, but his heart stopped as they were getting ready to transport, so they coded him all the way to the hospital.

When I went to examine the patient it was apparent we were unlikely to resuscitate him but since the paramedics had started we gave it a try. As we were working, the chest surgeon was passing the ER and he asked if he could try open heart massage. I saw no reason not to because we were getting nowhere, so he opened the chest and started, but it was apparent there was no blood. The only fluid to leak out was clear IV fluid. The patient had totally exsanguinated on scene. Further exam showed the knife had hit one of the great vessels in the chest from the back.

I read that one historian had said that people who were malcontents kept moving west until they fetched up against the Pacific and there they had to stop. That explained why so many strange people lived there. One lady I saw in the ER had been beaten by her boyfriend, and after sewing her lacerations, I talked with her about abusive relationships. She told me she didn't know where to go because she had moved to California from Nevada to escape another abusive boyfriend. It became readily apparent she picked guys who were abusive, so I sent her on to the counseling unit at the county psychiatric clinic, but history suggests there was little likelihood they would be able to help her. Women who pick such abusive boyfriends seem to continue to pick such men.

We had minimal backup in the smaller hospital I worked in and sometimes none at all. One night a family brought in their eleven-year-old girl with low abdominal pain. Exam and lab were suggestive of appendicitis but not diagnostic. Today we would do a helical CT and know what was going on, but in those days the accepted method was to watch the child for twelve to twenty-four hours and see which way the blood count and exam went. I called the local surgeon and he refused to come in and see the child so I had to call the surgeon in my town and have the family drive sixty miles in the middle of the night to see a surgeon. The surgeon in my hometown watched the girl overnight, and by morning she was doing much better so he released her. There was quite an uproar over this since it turned out the girl's father was on the county board of supervisors. I could see both sides since it was a great inconvenience to transfer a patient so far, but on the other hand if the surgeon had been too sleep deprived already, would you want him making decisions about your kid?

One of the ugliest cases I encountered was brought in by the police. This was a brother and sister who were at the beach and she was accusing him of rape. When I talked to her, she said this wasn't the first time, and she had decided to finally press charges. I went ahead and got out a "rape kit," which was supplied by the state for such circumstances. The rape kit is similar to what you see on CSI. We would take both vaginal and rectal swabs and then brush the pubic hair to catch any fibers or foreign hairs. We would do a drawing of any bruises or lacerations and take a Polaroid of any lesions as well. We would also cut a sample of pubic hair. I finished doing the kit on the young woman and started another on her brother who was passed out drunk. It was readily apparent he had recently had sex, and we did all the same things and both kits were sealed and signed by me and given to the police officer. I later learned that just as had apparently happened in the past when everybody sobered up, the charges were dropped, and I suspect the scenario was just going to repeat itself over and over. That's one of the reasons the cops aren't very impressed with charges of rape. My first Ob-Gyn partner had worked while getting his MPH by doing rape kits at Oakland General Hospital, and he said of the hundreds he'd done, he only had to testify in court once. For a variety of reasons most of these cases get dropped.

One of our regulars in the newer ER was a fellow who would come in asking for pain drugs every Friday night. He would claim severe tooth pain and tell the doc he just needed enough to get through to Tuesday when he had a dental appointment. This guy had a chart the size of a New York phone book, and it was full of identical ER visits. He did have terrible teeth with some of them rotted all the way to the gum line. In spite of that he never got them fixed because he would lose his pass to the ER. I usually sent him out with the recommendation he get some oil of cloves at the drugstore and apply it to the teeth that were hurting. That would give temporary relief, but I doubt he ever used it.

Small ERs are a challenge because the backup is minimal at best and may take some time to arrive. Sometimes you end up doing things you didn't know you could do because if you didn't no one would. Unfortunately you also are living on adrenalin and that probably isn't a good idea.

The University

After several months of looking, I found an ad for a job in the Health Service at a Midwestern university that was close to Susan's home, and since she still had relatives in the area, she was more amenable to moving there. I called the director of the program and after a talk he offered to pay my way to come and interview. We flew in in a snowstorm and were put up in a hotel right next to campus. I met with both the program director and the medical director. The service was different in that they saw not only students but faculty and staff of the university as well. This had the advantage that I would be able to use more of my skills. I was also interviewed by several of the staff in a sort of rolling interview afternoon. The salary was less than I had been making, but considering that call consisted of answering the phone and not going in and there were no inpatient responsibilities, it seemed adequate especially when one looked at the benefits. I was growing older and my retirement plan was lousy. It seemed with six kids, there was always something we needed the money for other than retirement.

We were back home for two or three days when the director called and offered me the job. I still had the insurance tail problem, but they didn't need me for five months so I had to pay only one-sixth of the tail or about $10,000. My group agreed to take it out of what they owed me for my share of the corporation. We put our house on the market and soon had it sold at a fair price so everything was looking up. (I should have been suspicious.) I was chief of staff at our hospital that year, so I had to get the vice-chief to take over my last three months. Since Thanh was in college and Doug was in love, they elected to stay put, but the other four children moved with us. Doug had been living on his own for a while anyway, and we arranged for

Thanh to stay with my surgeon friend's family while going to the local college.

The move went fairly smoothly, and we shipped most of our books since book rate was cheaper. We had flown out a couple times to house hunt and found a beautiful Victorian farm house costing only about $80,000 more than we had hoped to pay. I got rid of a couple pickup trucks full of paperbacks to smooth the transition. I had one month's salary from the university for the move, and amazingly the cost came out almost exactly on the button (I suspected the trucker knew what was available and cheated just a little to let us get a little more on the truck).

When we moved into our new home, we were greeted by a note in the mailbox asking us to collect our books at the post office because they were crowding out the workers. We were sitting in our new living room that first week when we heard gun fire in our yard. This was a little disconcerting but turned out to be a sheriff trying to take care of a deer, which had been hit on the road and had a broken leg. The officer was a little lazy and was shooting out of his cruiser's window with a pistol. We had to get used to deer being hit out front because our property had an old apple orchard and across the road was a corn field so we were in deer heaven.

Working for the university was an entirely different experience. I was no longer the boss and was no longer known around town. The town was crawling with MDs and PhDs, some of whom were nationally known. My office was all set up for me by the secretary who worked on our floor, and she had all the forms I needed to function in a bureaucracy.

We had one nurse who worked for everybody on the floor, and I was assigned a nurse practitioner who reported to me. This lady was very well trained and really needed very little guidance. I quickly learned she would come to me with anything she was uncomfortable with. There was another physician and nurse practitioner on the floor as well. I was told when I was hired I was to be the senior physician on this floor, but everybody had been there much longer, and there really was no such position officially.

I had a week to get oriented and one day in the afternoon my immediate superior (the medical director) took me over to the hospital to orient me there even though we had no inpatient responsibilities. There was an afternoon thunderstorm forecast, and we both took umbrellas. When we were leaving the hospital, there was a lightning strike on a crane in the parking lot. We both were shocked by our umbrellas. He threw his reflexively, and I had a spark jump from the metal rod of the umbrella to my thumb, which went into spasm. He shouted good-bye as he ran for his car. I later delighted in telling everyone that my first week on the job my boss had tried to get me killed.

I was assigned to the general clinic four days a week, and one day was in the Gyn clinic. It quickly became apparent the Gyn clinic was a waste of time since most of the patients were young collage girls, and they didn't want a man doing their exams. I spent much of my time there doing nothing. I saw some patients, but they were somewhat grudgingly on my schedule only because all the women providers had full schedules. One such young woman filed a complaint because in an effort to get her to relax, I had tried to joke with her, and she complained that I was having way too much fun and must get my jollies from doing the exam. I eventually told the administration I would continue doing Gyn exams but only in my office as I had for nearly twenty years before coming to the university.

Early on I ran into one of the problems that were to plague me for the rest of my time at the university. I had a seventeen-year-old daughter of a faculty member brought in with an ankle injury. X-rays showed a fracture of one of the bones just above the ankle. This appeared to be slightly displaced, and that can be a problem. If the joint is misaligned, it will never work right so I wanted a second opinion from an orthopedic surgeon. I asked my colleagues how I did that, and they suggested I call the resident in Ortho who was on call. I did that and he told me to send her to the ER, and if they needed him, they would call him. I explained I didn't need an ER opinion but just an Ortho opinion, but he refused to be helpful. I talked to the chief resident in Ortho and got the same runaround. It happened the head of the department of Orthopedics was a friend of the orthopedic surgeon in my old town, and I'd been asked to say hello for him. I called the department head and said hi from his old friend and told him the problem I was having, and he said just to send the patient to the ER and his residents would be down immediately. That was what we did, and after a couple hours of hassle, three residents met her in the ER. It seemed the house staff had no way to see patients when their clinic wasn't running and really had no desire to see anyone anyway. The faculty were mostly willing to make arrangements if you knew them, but otherwise you had to send patients through an ER with as much as twelve-hour waits to get someone to agree with you and call the required specialist. Since they didn't always agree with you, sometimes, after all that wait, the patient was never seen by the specialist. This was a complete change since in private practice, the various specialists would be only too happy to see a patient if you asked them. Their income was dependent on referrals, and I also felt they just naturally felt more compassion than the residents who seemed to be mostly concerned about not working too hard.

I had one young African-American woman come in complaining of joint pain and stiffness and general malaise. Tiredness is a common complaint with students, and you often find they're trying to get by on six hours sleep when they need eight or nine or more at that age, but the joints were a whole new kettle of fish. I ran the usual tests for rheumatoid arthritis and lupus as well as parvovirus and found she was strongly positive for lupus antibodies. I started her on steroids and referred her to a rheumatologist at the university clinic who took care of nothing but lupus. I continued to care for her general needs for most of the rest of the time I worked at the university, even through two pregnancies. All in all she did very well with a disease we used to think was always terminal.

We pulled night call for a week at a time and received some additional compensation for doing so. When I first started, the night calls went to the nurse practitioners at the hospital, and they would handle most of them and call you for help or to let you know they'd had the patient come in to get evaluated. Unfortunately this didn't last long before the hospital wanted to charge us for the service, and the calls were moved to coming directly to us through an answering service. Since there was a mid-level (nurse-practitioner or physician's assistant) taking call for the student's part of the time, the answering service could never figure out whom to give the calls to. The physicians got all the calls after 10:00 p.m. and students didn't seem to call much before midnight anyway. The calls were much different from private practice. One call was especially common and that was "the condom broke, what do we do?" Since we didn't always have an all-night pharmacy and the students didn't always have transportation available, it saved me explaining I didn't do things which could cause fetal death and I could just have them come in to the clinic in the morning and see one of the clinicians who did prescribe "morning after pills."

In the summer the physicians pulled all the call since there were fewer students around. One evening my wife and I were at Sear's picking up a patio set we had ordered when I received a call from a young female student in a panic because she'd seen some blood in her stool. I was sympathetic with her being upset and explained to her that the amount wasn't enough to worry about and that red blood in the stool of someone her age usually meant either a small hemorrhoid or a small tear in the rectal skin. I suggested she come to clinic in the morning and we would look, but in the meantime she shouldn't worry. That explanation seemed to satisfy her but then she said "Oh, while I have you on the line, sometimes my butt crack itches." I explained to her that I wasn't going to discuss her itchy butt crack while sitting in Sear's parking lot, but she could ask when she came to the clinic the next morning. My wife was laughing herself silly listening to this conversation.

The students weren't very medically sophisticated and carried misinformation with them from their parents or their physicians at home. One of the big problems we faced was the absolute belief that they wouldn't get well unless they were given an antibiotic for what was an obvious viral illness for which an antibiotic is useless and really contraindicated. As our director was fond of saying, we practiced in a fish bowl, meaning everything we did was scrutinized by parents and home physicians so we had to be very careful what we said. One young lady came in to be seen because she'd had a cold for six weeks, and her mother (a general practitioner elsewhere) had had her on a very powerful antibiotic and she wasn't getting better. I explained to her that I thought they had proven this illness wasn't going to respond to antibiotics, and we went with cold medications and tested her for mononucleosis which she had.

The faculty often knew just enough to get into trouble. One of my first encounters with a professor I later came to know rather well occurred when he came to my office with a rather minor problem and dropped on my desk about a hundred-page literature search from the medical library on the treatment of his problem. He pointed to a couple articles and said he wanted a prescription for that drug. I had to tell him I couldn't give it to him, and when he got somewhat huffy and wanted to know why not, I had to point out these were research articles and the FDA hadn't approved that drug for use yet. I went ahead and prescribed something that was approved, and since it worked fine he never brought a literature search to my office again although I think he still frequently ran them anyway.

Over time I gradually collected a group of faculty on my patient panel, some of which were from the medical school. I had one young medical student sent to me because he just wasn't feeling well. Initial exam wasn't helpful but I ran a group of screening tests and found his sedimentation rate ran off the charts. This is a simple test that responds to the presence of inflammation anywhere in the body, but it was very unusual to see it so high in a young person. A chest x-ray revealed a mass in the middle of the chest where there are many lymph nodes. I got hold of one of the oncology surgeons to biopsy the mass, and unfortunately it turned out to be a non-Hodgkin's lymphoma. The young man was immediately started on radiation and chemotherapy, and after two years was able to return to medical school as well as his PhD program (he was doing a combined program), and as long as I knew him, he stayed disease free.

Early on we had a procedure room that was curtained off into cubicles and that was where we did minor procedures. Because of my ER and surgical background, I was sent a lot of the cases that were going to require some sort of intervention. One such case got us a new set of curtains. This young man came in with a large boil on his back, and when I went to drain it, it was under pressure and shot pus and blood onto the curtains. When we had packed the abscess, my nurse contacted housekeeping to get the drapes cleaned, but the head of the building services refused and had us simply throw the drapes away and bought us new ones.

I had one very sad case of a thirty-two-year-old graduate student who came to see me for a second opinion. She had noticed a breast lump several months earlier and had come into Gynecology to have it checked. The chief of Gynecology saw her and arranged a needle biopsy. This was reported to show only some inflammation but no malignant cells. She was still worried and came to see me. I saw her just before Christmas, and my exam made me very uncomfortable. I suggested getting at least a mammogram and probably an open biopsy. She wanted to know if it could wait a couple weeks until the New Year when her grad student insurance would kick in. I was a little uncomfortable with this, but she had had a negative biopsy, and we decided two weeks probably weren't going to change anything. Right after New Year's we got her mammogram and I immediately got a call from the radiologist at the breast clinic who told me she didn't care what the needle biopsy said; this was cancer. That being the case I had the breast surgeons see her and they arranged to do an open lumpectomy and lymph node dissection of the arm pit to check for metastasis. The surgery found cancer but the lymph nodes were all clear so we were hopeful she would be fine with just the lumpectomy. A few weeks later, I got a call from her oncologic surgeon that she hadn't been feeling well, and her liver seemed enlarged so they had scanned her and found her liver was full of metastases. With her lymph nodes negative, this was very unusual but could happen. We discussed this with the oncologist, and she was started on chemotherapy but the outlook wasn't good. Finally they contacted me and suggested she needed to find a bone marrow donor.

The thinking at that time was that if you did heavy-duty chemotherapy, you could kill all the cancer cells but you would kill out the bone marrow and then you could save the patient by replacing her bone marrow with a transplant. The cost for this procedure was around $100,000 and the insurance refused to pay. This was a very difficult situation because the insurance company was owned by the university. The university oncologists were saying it was her only chance and the university insurance was saying it was experimental and they weren't paying for it. I became something of an irritant at the insurance company, and they finally resolved it by finding a researcher on campus who had a grant to study this procedure. He agreed to include her in his study, which meant the procedure was paid for by his grant.

The patient finally underwent the chemo and had the bone marrow transplant, but a short time later, the liver lesions returned. It was apparent we had done everything science knew how to do, and she went home to her parents where she eventually expired. At this time this procedure has been shown not to work, but I would have felt terrible if we hadn't tried everything we thought at the time might work. I didn't feel so good about the whole case as it was.

A major source of injuries on campus was the loft. These were add-ons that were sold to the students to help with their small dorm rooms. They were essentially the upper bunk bed that could be built over the standard bed in the room. Students were constantly falling out of them, only sometimes because they weren't sober. Missed steps, bad dreams, and simply forgetting they were in a loft and stepping out in the morning all contributed to the number of injuries we saw. Because of my ER background I was frequently asked to see these injuries. One young lady hit a glass shelf on the way down and skinned her nose, leaving a roll of skin on the bridge. It was full thickness and was obviously going to leave a scar. I advised her that it needed to be fixed, and either she could trust me to do it or we could send her to the ER and see if they would get a facial plastics specialist or just decide to fix it themselves. She elected to have me do it, so I got out my special magnifying glasses and was able to unroll the skin and line it up with where it had been. I tacked it into place with some very fine suture and held the middle of the flap down with a cotton bolster, which I tied into place with suture thereby pushing the center of the flap down in the center to hopefully get a blood supply. It healed very nicely and she left for the summer but came back in the fall as I'd asked to show me the results. You really couldn't see where the flap had come down. I always worried a little when I did one of these more difficult cases because if it ended up in court, I really didn't have the credentials that would protect me.

One such case occurred a few years later when I had a young lady who had fallen and sustained a cut just under her chin. This is a very common injury in the ER, and I had no qualms about fixing it although with young ladies' faces I tend to be very careful anyway. Apparently after she got back to her dorm, she called her mother who called my secretary and screamed into the phone to get that f—ing doctor on the phone. When she was told I was gone to lunch she continued to scream that she wanted those f—ing stitches removed and she wanted a plastic surgeon to take care of her daughter. Later she called back and apparently had called a local plastics man who told her not to have the stitches removed (I wouldn't have removed them anyway since that's an almost sure way to get an infection). She told us she hoped for our sakes we hadn't ruined her daughter's modeling career. I was a little surprised by that since I had seen her daughter and hadn't even remotely suspected she had a great modeling career ahead of her. Things healed well, and I guess the scar wasn't too bad because I never heard from her again.

Many people don't understand that the primary consideration in repairing a wound is to get it closed and healed without an infection. If you follow certain principles, you may minimize the scarring. The time to really deal with a scar is after everything's healed when you can make a clean incision without foreign bodies, and tissue transfers are much less likely to get infected. The sooner a wound is closed, the better your chances of getting a good result. Many people won't close a wound older than twelve hours although that really doesn't hold with the face, which has a good blood supply and can usually be closed late if the wound isn't grossly contaminated.

I had one young lady come in with a lesion on her cheek, which was highly suspicious for melanoma, a deadly skin cancer. She wanted it removed even though I warned her it could leave a scar, which would be hard to hide. We could biopsy it and see if it had to go, but she felt a scar would be less disfiguring than the lesion was.

I agreed to schedule her and spent some time figuring out how to align my incision to cause the least visible scarring. People often don't realize that when you cut skin, you always get at least some scar, and the trick is to hide it in the regular skin lines we have all over our bodies. With this lesion I also wanted at least a couple millimeters margins in case it was melanoma. I knew that would be inadequate if it was cancerous, but I was hoping for the best. With great care the skin came together looking very good, but unfortunately the biopsy was reported as superficial, spreading melanoma with clear margins. I sent her to the Melanoma Clinic where (as I knew they would) they recommended wider margins and called in facial plastics to help the oncological surgeon with the excision. They did a beautiful job, but I was a little down that after all my work they had to excise what I thought would be a nice scar. The young woman had the most remarkable attitude, and as far as I know was lesion free as long as she was at the university. Unfortunately about 20 percent of these lesions will regrow, so she needed to be watched for life.

One of the interesting things at the university was the number of foreign students and faculty. I had one man brought in from the business school in obvious pain. He was there for a short course to upgrade his skills in business. His friend and interpreter told me he was in pain from a self-administered circumcision. I had never heard of such a thing, but his friend showed me the instructions that came with a kit. It seems that the Asian businessmen had noted that most American businessmen were circumcised, and they wanted to look the same, for reasons I never could fathom. These kits were sold over the counter and consisted of a bell-like plastic piece that went over the glans, and the foreskin was stretched over this. Then a ligature was tied around the base tightly to cut off the blood supply to the foreskin, which was supposed to drop off. His knot left a tiny place for blood to reach a tiny portion of the foreskin, which was still alive and really hurt. I injected a little local to his great relief and cut the tiny piece of foreskin off and cauterized the base so it wouldn't bleed. He left much happier than when he had come in.

The foreign students often had no understanding of the availability of medical care in the United States. One night we had closed up and were getting ready to go home when we hear a banging on the front door. My nurse went down to see what was going on and found a group of Asian students standing outside supporting a young girl who appeared to be approaching unconsciousness. They brought her in, and we discovered we could palpate (feel) a blood pressure at about fifty but couldn't hear one at all. The story was that this girl had had severe diarrhea for three days and didn't know what to do, so she stayed in her dorm room for the whole time not eating or drinking anything. This girl couldn't have weighed a hundred pounds before she got sick. When she could no longer stand up, one of her friends knew about the health service but none of them knew about ERs or 911. If they had been five minutes later, we would probably have found a dead girl on our front porch in the morning. As it was, I got an IV into her to pour in the fluids while we waited for the ambulance, which took her to the university hospital ER. She did fine of course once she was rehydrated.

A similar incident occurred one Saturday morning. We had walk-in clinic on Saturday from nine to noon on Saturdays. We locked the door at noon and stayed until all the patients who were waiting got seen. As we were closing up, I heard banging on the front door and looked out to see an Asian woman crying and very upset. She told me she and her husband had come from Seattle to see their son graduate from business school. He'd turned up that morning dressed in suit and tie but insisted on going out in the street to hand out slips of paper with gibberish on them. I walked out into the street and talked him into coming inside and sitting with his parents. We called the campus police to transport him to the psych ER by force if necessary although he turned out to be very co-operative. Two days later his parents turned up in my clinic to thank us for getting him the help he needed. Fortunately he was having a manic episode and therefore was very treatable as opposed to a schizophrenic break, which wouldn't be as treatable. They also brought me rice balls for lunch, which was great. About a year later I heard from the son that he had a very responsible job with a Fortune 500 company and was well controlled with medication.

Another person with psychiatric problems didn't turn out so well. I had seen this girl several times for various problems and had noted a very strange personality. She was a first year medical student and presumably had been thoroughly screened before being admitted to medical school, though in this case apparently not enough. She came in one day and told me she had a very sore throat. She'd started with a standard sore throat but reasoned that if she could kill the virus she'd get over it faster so she tried to gargle boiling water. She had first and second degree burns of her mouth and throat. Fortunately these had not swelled enough to interfere with breathing and had been there since the night before, so all I could recommend was cool saline (salt water) swishes and pain medication. Fortunately our consulting psychiatrist was also the psychiatrist assigned to the medical students, so I could call her and warn her about this girl. I never saw the girl again.

After I'd been at the university for a while, my boss asked if I was interested in teaching. There was a class in physical diagnosis that needed volunteers to help out, and the boss said I could go one afternoon a week as part of my duties. I agreed and started working the class. There were two parts to the class. Part one was with the first year students and consisted of teaching exam techniques. The professor would have people with different problems come in, and the students would examine a patient while I observed their technique. I elected to do the pulmonary section, and there were about five or six instructors each with a patient with chronic pulmonary problems to demonstrate the various findings. Groups of four or five students would rotate to the various patients. This seemed very stressful for the students, but they almost always got the exam right even if they couldn't always use the data to make a diagnosis.

The second part of the class occurred in the second year when we were assigned two students, and every week we would take them to the university hospital where they had a patient to take a history and do a physical on. The patients were all volunteers, and most were very patient although not all of them understood what they had volunteered for.

One day I was with my students when a man with a large entourage came up to me in the hallway and wanted to know where my name tag was. I pointed to the name tag I always wore, and he got very sarcastic and told me in front of my students and all his sycophants that I had to get my university tag on or he'd get me fired. He then walked away looking very proud of himself. I asked one of his followers who he was, and she told me he was the top boss. I'd had one other run-in with this fool, and this time I planned to file a formal complaint. He never knew there were physicians in the university who weren't under his control, but in fact I worked under a different division. Unfortunately this occurred on a Friday, and the paper the next morning said he'd been fired by the president. I felt bad she'd gotten to him before my complaint, so I couldn't take any credit for his firing.

Early in my time at the university I had a young lady come in very sick with obvious jaundice and a severe sore throat. She was from Sweden and had only come for a six-week course at the business school. She'd barely arrived in this country when her symptoms began, and the school directed her to Health Service. Since she was from Sweden and only going to be here a few weeks, she had not thought to get insurance. She was having difficulty keeping even fluids down, and I would have preferred to hospitalize her but she refused. The laboratory studies came back positive for mono hepatitis, which is a form of infectious mononucleosis involving the liver. I actually talked with her father in Sweden. He was a physician there and spoke very good English. I outlined my treatment plans for her, and he said that's exactly what they'd do in Sweden. I would rehydrate her every day in our observation area and had started her on steroids, which can make remarkable reversible of the symptoms in mono. I talked to her father nearly daily. By bringing her in and rehydrating her every day, we got her under control. When the nausea settled down, we arranged for her to go back to Sweden for the rest of her convalescence. She was terribly disappointed she'd missed her class and never saw anything of America except Health Service and her dorm room.

A lady who was on the university staff came in one day with a huge bruise on her head, which she alleged was the result of abuse by her boyfriend. She said she was having dizzy spells, and although her exam was normal, I sent her for a CT of the head. The CT report was very strange because they reported a mass just beneath the bruise but said it was a growth and not from trauma. This seemed to me to be very unlikely, so I had an MRI done but got the same report. I sent her along to the neurosurgeons with some trepidation, but in fact they ended up removing a small meningioma (benign brain tumor) from her head and she did well after. I wonder how big this mass would have gotten if our attention hadn't been called to her head by her abusive boyfriend.

It seemed that all my life I'd been looking for an acoustic neuroma with no luck until a former secretary of mine who had moved on in the university came in complaining of dizziness and buzzing in her ear. I was suspicious and got an audiogram. Our audiologist felt the pattern in that ear was compatible with acoustic neuroma (Schwannoma of the eighth nerve). CT of the area confirmed the diagnosis, and I sent her on to the ENT surgeons who were able to remove it without affecting her hearing. I was pleased when they told her it was one of the smallest they'd seen.

Most of the physicians in the Health Service had never been in private practice and had never had the pressure of seeing patients at a rapid clip in order to pay the bills. My colleague on the third floor tried to keep up with me, and even though he was an excellent physician, he became very frustrated when he did. When we surveyed we found that most of my patients were seen early or on time, which gave me the freedom to work in extra patients when needed.

There was an older FP on the first floor who had done most of the procedures, and when he retired, I would do most of them although I told everyone I would be glad to train them. The procedure most needed was opening abscesses including pilonidal abscesses, which are common at the age of college students. I operate under the old saw that you should "never let the sun set on an abscess." I could see no reason why a patient should be sent home to suffer while waiting for a space in the schedule. I also had some trouble convincing some of my colleagues that the treatment of an abscess is drainage, not antibiotics.

We had several specialty clinics available including Dermatology, Neurology, Optometry, Audiology, ENT, and Orthopedics. We also had a few problems for which we didn't have good coverage. One of the major problem areas was feet. The students and some of the faculty and staff had a fair number of foot problems. One of the major sources of these problems was the marching band, which, when I came, was using a rapid high step march, which was really hard on the feet. Since most musicians weren't in top shape anyway, we would begin to see foot problems about a week before the fall semester when the band arrived early to begin practicing for football season. It was considered a great honor to play in the football band, so the kids would push themselves when they shouldn't, and even when they had a stress fracture would beg me to let them march. I got a couple of podiatric textbooks and read them cover to cover and eventually worked up a lecture on sore feet for the rest of Health Service.

One of the problems that was very common among the students was ingrown toenails especially on the great toe. Most of these seemed to relate to picking or cutting the toenails like a fingernail. Often the solution was just to put a little cotton under the in grown nail to allow it to grow out over the skin and then start cutting it square across so the skin did not come up in front of the growing nail when they put weight on it. Interestingly, one of my daughters was in college elsewhere and had that problem. She called me to complain that the doctor there had told her about the cotton, and she felt he was just a quack. I told her I was glad they had someone who knew what to do. I do wonder how many of my patients called their parents with the same complaint.

Some of the nails were so bad either because of anatomy or chronicity they would require surgical revision. The older way was to remove the side of the nail that was in-growing and to destroy the bed with phenol, which is a terribly caustic substance. The rule had been that if you want to do that, you had to go to the Health Service Pharmacy and carry the stuff to your procedure room yourself because the pharmacist wouldn't carry it around the building. But right after I started we got a machine that used radar frequency to cut tissue and was used for cervical biopsy in the Gyn clinic. This machine had a special tip, which would fit into the corner of the nail matrix and destroy the nail-forming cells. It was nontoxic and much more reliable then phenol so I began using it with great success.

Because the neurology clinic was held in the evening and the full lab wasn't there, they had a problem when they needed a lumbar puncture for diagnosis of things like MS. Since this was an age group in which the initial diagnosis was usually made, the neurologists saw a fair number of these. They started sending these patients in to see me the next day for their lumbar puncture, which was good for me since I got to do enough to keep my skills up.

As time went along, I was asked if I could teach residents as the senior residents in Family Medicine had a couple of electives and one was interested in Health Service. Although there had been a ban on residents out of fears of anonymity problems with the students, the boss gave me the green light and I scheduled the young man who had asked.

One patient I had inherited when I came had poorly controlled adult diabetes, and I had tried to get him under much better control, but I was probably too late. He came in one day when my resident was there so I had the resident do his history and physical. The patient's only complaint was that he would get dizzy and lose his balance. When I went in to check the resident's findings, he said he didn't think the patient was really dizzy but he had lost proprioception in his feet (the ability to tell where your feet are). And his feet were going numb. Even with the help of the Diabetes Clinic at the university, this patient proceeded to almost every complication you can get from diabetes including needing a four-vessel coronary artery bypass and getting a renal transplant. His foot problems progressed to the point he had to also have an amputation. Only his eyes were spared the last time I saw him. He was a lay minister in a local black church and was always smiling and never complained. But he did have to give up his job at the university.

That resident had his sister rotate with me the next year and the last I heard about him he was the director of a health service in a prominent university. His sister was my wife's primary physician for years.

The boss called me in one day to tell me that the physician who had been our Communicative Disorders Clinic liaison would be leaving to go back to training. He asked if I would take the position. This clinic was run by the Speech Pathology Department and had to have an MD as a medical director. This clinic brought people in from all over the country to relearn speech after brain injury such as stroke or traumatic damage. My job would primarily consist of supplying needed medical care such as monitoring blood thinners and blood pressure medications. I agreed and asked if I could put Medical Director of CDC on my business card, but he thought that was a little much. The result of this was that I got to meet people from all over the country, including a couple famous actors. Some of the cases were very sad such as the lady lawyer who at thirty-five had a stroke while delivering her child and the forty-year-old woman who was a professor of piano at a nearby university whose left side wouldn't work after a stroke.

One duty I was asked to perform was to give a lecture about stroke at an annual luncheon held for the families of the patients for that year.

The luncheon was interrupted by the Director of Health Care (see above) who came through with an entourage and introduced himself to everyone telling them that he was in charge of all health care on campus. The clinic was under speech pathology, and I was under Student Services, and nobody there was under his division except the stroke expert from Neurology. Some egos are amazing.

After I had been at the university for several years, the physician in charge of our continuing education course decided to leave and I was asked to take over. My nurse practitioner and I began scheduling lectures. The course consisted of a one-hour lecture weekly on various subjects of interest to outpatient medicine specialists as well as updates on current practice in the specialties. This had two advantages for me in that I could schedule subjects I was interested in, and I got to know many of the hospital specialists I might otherwise not have run into. Since I had no budget, I had to use the university's specialists who were expected to supply the university with such talks as part of their salaries. I soon developed a stable of regulars who seemed to enjoy the talks and were good speakers. Many of these physicians were used to giving update talks to various courses the university ran for the community and for their residents and therefore only had to modify something they had already worked out.

Shortly after fall semester started, one eighteen-year-old male came into my office in a state of panic because his genitals had swollen to nearly twice normal size. His story was that he'd been in the Central Campus Recreational Building for three days working out since he'd never had access to such facilities at home. When he was changing, he'd noted the swelling. When I examined him, he was massively swollen to the point you could nearly read newsprint through the skin. I ordered some stat labs but had no idea what he'd done, and we were closing so I called the chief of the ER at the university who happened to be working that shift and told him what I was dealing with. We agreed I would transfer the youngster to the ER, and the chief would pick up the case and see if he could work out what had happened. The next day I got a call from the ER chief to tell me the youngster had a CK (a muscle enzyme, which is normally inside the cell) of over seventeen thousand. This indicates massive muscle damage.

Apparently the young man had exercised so much that he'd injured a lot of muscles especially in the abdomen. The genital swelling was just the result of the swelling from the injured muscle settling into the lowest and loosest tissue. The real concern was myoglobin, which is released when muscle is broken down and can clog the kidney tubules, so we had him come in two or three days in a row to check his urine, but it always stayed normal.

The young men had their own problems, which included STDs (sexually transmitted diseases), prostatitis and epididymitis, testicular cancer, and torsioned testicle (testicle twisted on its blood supply). One young man came in complaining of severe pain in a testicle, and my resident saw him. The differential was between torsion and epididymitis, and I felt he had epididymitis probably because of his prostate tenderness. We started him on pain meds and antibiotics, but things didn't get better and he went to the ER where they diagnosed torsion and sent him to surgery where the testicle was judged too far gone and it was removed. This condition needs surgery within three hours to have any chance of saving the testicle. I felt very badly that I missed it although we still may not have saved the testicle anyway, and most men do fine with only one. A few months later when I was sued it was the only time when I felt the plaintiff deserved some compensation, but the case was thrown out of court because I was a state employee and couldn't be sued (that was later changed by the legislature).

There is an entity called intermittent torsion where the torsion comes and goes with movement. I had one young man come in with torsion by exam and history and immediately sent him to the ER and advised the urologist on call he was coming. By the time he got to the ER, the torsion had relieved itself, and they apparently didn't believe he had been torsioned. They sent him out, and a couple days later he came in with the same problem. Fearing another de-torsion on the way to the ER, I did an ultrasound at Health Service, which showed the torsion and also showed it de-torsioned a few minutes later. I sent him back to the ER, and they got him an appointment in Urology clinic several days later. When he went to clinic, he was seen by a urologist who specialized in prostate cancer and was not impressed. The young man came back to me very upset because he had no insurance and was receiving $17,000 in bills with nothing being done. It happened I knew the chief of urology who was a very compassionate guy, and I called him and told him the story. He saw the patient himself and scheduled and did his surgery. I also gave the patient the name of the person in the loss prevention office who could fix his bill and I hope that worked.

Chronic prostatitis was a constant problem because it was very difficult to treat and could be caused by numerous organisms. Young men with burning urination almost never had a urinary infection, and the other symptoms such as back or groin ache were quite non-specific. Because the cause of this problem could be bacterial or viral (or even mycoplasmal, an organism in between) and the methods to identify the organism were so poor, we would usually just treat with antibiotics blindly and hope they worked. Since we generally did not know the organism, if the patient did not improve, we would try a second antibiotic, and if that didn't help, we'd use anti-inflammatories. Usually about that point the patient was losing faith in me, so I would send him to urology clinic just to make him feel we'd tried everything. Most of the time they'd tell him we were doing what could be done. That didn't necessarily make a happy patient, but at least they began to understand.

Testicular cancer is a disease of young men and therefore was a constant worry. We tried to get young men to do self-exam just as the women were taught breast self-exam. When they found a lump most of them would arrive in the office in a state of panic. Right behind the testicle is the epididymis, which will form cysts, and most of the time that is what they were finding, but early in my time at the university, I had a seventeen-year-old freshman who had a testicular cancer both by exam and by ultrasound. He had no evidence of spread and was sent to urology where it was immediately removed. I don't remember if he had any chemotherapy or not, but he did well.

Later in my time at the university I had a young man come in with mild testicular pain and a cough. He told me the painful testicle had been in his abdomen at birth and was later surgically brought down into the scrotum. The reason the testicle is brought down is the increased temperature from being in the abdomen makes cancer of the testicle much more likely. He'd seen his own physician in a nearby suburb and was told there was an abnormality on the ultrasound, but they thought it was from the previous surgery. Exam of his scrotum did feel strange but not diagnostic. His lungs however had strange wheezes and we did a chest x-ray that showed "puff balls" all over his lungs. The radiologist called me and said he didn't know anything in this age group that would look like that except metastatic testicular cancer. We went ahead and did an ultrasound of the scrotum and found a mass compatible with cancer. I hated to interfere with his relationship with his own physician, but I wasn't really impressed with the diagnostic acumen. I gave him the choice of returning to his physician or going to the university ER with his x-rays and ultrasound and notes from the radiologist and myself as to what we thought was happening. He wanted to go to his physician. This was a Friday but his physician had Saturday office hours, so I called and talked with one of the physicians in the office, and they got him on the schedule for the next morning. Later I learned he had talked it over with his parents and decided to go to the ER after all. I saw they had started his chemotherapy in the ER. He responded so well he was back in class in couple weeks getting his chemotherapy as an outpatient. This is one cancer with which we get excellent results. When he had no-showed at his doctor's office Saturday morning, they had not been concerned. I had tracked him down because I was so worried about him.

The university environment takes some getting used to. You are more likely to get in trouble for not being politically correct than for doing a poor job. I had one young man come in and tell me how he was chewed out by a woman he was helping load her car at a local store where he worked. It was a few days before Christmas, and as he finished, he wished her a Merry Christmas. Apparently she became very angry and screamed at him much to his confusion.

Shortly after I arrived, my boss knew I was singing with the Cantata Singers and had told people in the administration about it. They wanted a group to carol at the annual holiday party, which was decorated with a holiday tree and a little village. I agreed and went to a short rehearsal of this caroling quartet. They had only a few songs and there were things like "Jingle Bell Rock." I asked about singing real carols and was informed we couldn't sing anything with the word

"Christmas" in it because we might offend someone. I pointed out that was my holiday and I was offended by such an attitude. The point to me was that this is a holiday that is near Hanukah and Kwanza, and they could certainly be included but it was not a holiday for Muslims, Buddhists, Hindus, and many of the numerous other religions on campus. It seemed silly to call it a "holiday party" and even sillier to refer to a "holiday tree."

Since the students paid nothing for their visits, we were able to practice a better form of medicine on occasion. For example, if a student came in with one of the many sprained ankles we saw each day, we could bring them in daily either to our nurses or to PT to get their ankle re-taped. This is the most effective support available but seldom used because it's too expensive in other circumstances, so elastic braces are frequently used in ERs and private practice. We did have one student show up at four thirty on Friday afternoon, asking to get his ankles taped because he had an intermural basketball game that night. We taught him how to tape his own ankles and told him not to return except for medical care.

The faculty all have their own drummers, and since most of them are on tenure, they can pretty much do as they please. One young professor told me he always arranged his classes so he could be on the handball court by two every afternoon. I had one faculty member who always smelled so bad my nurses would complain. He was from a country where women stayed in their places and was always very nasty to my receptionist. I finally did have to speak to him about that.

One day I called a patient from the waiting room and was surprised to have a woman who looked like a bag-lady off the street come in. We dealt with her problem, but I wanted to see her back the next week. She asked if it would be OK if it was the week after as she had to be out of town the next week. I asked what she was doing, and she told me she had to lead a section of the National Science Association. It turned out she was world famous in her field.

In the summer we would get calls from students who had gone home but didn't know who to call when they got into trouble. One such student called me on a Sunday afternoon and asked what I knew about rabies. I asked why he wanted to know, and he related the bizarre story that he had seen a raccoon in his parent's back yard and it appeared to be ill. He'd inserted a tube down the animal's throat and tried to breath for it by mouth to tube. The animal died anyway, and after thinking about it afterward, he concluded the animal might have had rabies. He wanted to know if he got some saliva in his mouth and it had rabies, could he catch it. He'd called the local Health Department but they weren't open on Sunday afternoon. I suspected it never occurred to them they needed to stay open because somebody might be that dumb. I advised him he probably could get rabies that way and that he needed to put the body in a garbage bag and put it in his mother's freezer (hey, it's her kid) and on Monday morning he needed to be at the Health Department when they opened so they could have the brain checked for rabies. It turned out the animal had died of rabies, and we gave him the last two shots of his six-shot series when he got back to school in the fall.

Sometimes when you think you've done everything right, Murphy of Murphy's Law intervenes and the outcome can be terrible. I had a very obese diabetic lady whose knees were going out. We tried everything including steroid injections into the knee joints, which made her diabetes even harder to control. She had reached the point she could only get around using a walker and going three or four steps at a time and then having to rest. She seemed incapable of staying on a diet and very soon wasn't going to be able to work. The university hospital had recently started a bariatric surgery program, and she seemed to me to fit all their criteria so we discussed that. She thought about it and decided to consider it further. They required psych testing before they would consider her, and she went through it without problems. This patient had had leg clots and was on anticoagulants, which minimally complicated the surgery, but they routinely just stopped her medication long enough for it to wear off. Many programs would put a screen in the vena cava to prevent clots from getting to the lungs but they did not.

She underwent the surgery without problems and was recuperating when she started to bleed because they had restarted her anticoagulant and apparently overdid it. She went to the ER and was readmitted because of her hemorrhaging and given medication to reverse her anticoagulants. Shortly thereafter she clotted in her legs, threw a clot to her lungs, (pulmonary embolism), and died. It's hard not to feel you had some responsibility when something like that happens, but I really think the referral was appropriate if the management was less than stellar.

I was in my office one day when I got a phone call from Radiology that they needed me to come down stat (drop everything and run.) This was somewhat unusual, so I ran down to find a man obviously severely short of breath. The story was that he was playing volleyball when he felt a sudden sharp pain in his chest and became short of breath. The man had seen another physician in the building, and that physician thought he might have had a pneumothorax. This condition occurs when a weak part of the lung pops and leaks air into the space outside the lung but inside the lining around the lung. This causes the lung to collapse. I looked at the x-rays and this man's heart was moving to the wrong side of his chest so he had a thing called a tension pneumothorax where a one-way valve was formed by the rupture causing pressure to build up in the pneumothorax. This is extremely dangerous and must be treated immediately because every breath the patient took made the tension worse. We didn't have chest tubes like I would use in the ER, so I got the largest venous catheter we stocked and stuck that into the patient's chest. The pressure didn't equalize as it should have so I put a 50 cc syringe on the catheter and sucked the air out of the chest. As soon as that was done, the patient was able to breathe easier. Initially I had thought the patient was dark complected, but he turned pink as I removed the pressure. The pressure had been trapping the venous blood by twisting the return flow to the heart causing him to turn dark. We taped the catheter in place and showed the EMTs on the ambulance how to relieve the pressure should it start to build up again and sent him off to the ER. I suspect the ER docs had a laugh at my Jerry-rigged chest tube, but it worked and I suspect saved the man's life.

I had a Chinese grad student and his wife come into my office one day with the story that her father was in China and had chronic Hepatitis B, which is very common there. He was having trouble with liver failure, and they needed albumin to treat him but there was no albumin available in China. They wanted to know if they could buy some here and take it to him. I contacted our chief pharmacist and she agreed to order some from the hospital if I would write the prescription. We got ten 25 gram vials, and both the pharmacist and I wrote letters explaining the situation so we hoped the lady could get it through TSA. I later found out they did let it through, and she took it to China where they used it on her father who eventually got out of the hospital. When she came back, she brought me a small good luck charm made of jade, and the couple invited my wife and me out for dinner. They took us to a Chinese restaurant where they ordered from a Chinese menu (I didn't know they had two menus). I don't know what we had but it sure was good. I suppose that was a violation of the university policy of not taking gifts, but it was relatively minor and I certainly didn't want to cause them any loss of face by refusing their gift of gratitude.

Alcohol was a big problem on campus and was worse because many of the students didn't see it as a problem. I had one student brought in on a Saturday morning because a janitor thought he'd injured the kid because he hit him in the head when he opened a door behind which the student was passed out. He was obviously still inebriated at ten the next morning. We kept him under observation for the next couple hours, and I had a talk with him about binge drinking before he left. I also referred him to our alcohol counselor. He assured me he had to drink heavily because he was in a frat house, and it was expected. Later I was contacted by another member of our staff about this same young man who didn't remember being in to see me nor did he remember anything I had told him.

Saint Patrick's Day was always a problem. The bars would open at 7:00 a.m., and some of the students felt it was their obligation to get blind drunk. I always kind of wondered what the good saint would think of celebrating his day in that way.

While our clientele had many fewer drug seeking types than the ER, we also had physicians who weren't attuned to the problem. I saw one woman when her regular doc wasn't available, and she wanted a refill of her Vicodan. She lived in a nearby city and drove fifty miles to get this medication. She had a sallow complexion and very thick chart full of things for which she needed narcotics. I confronted her with her addiction and she admitted to me that she was even going to Canada where she could get 15 mg codeine and Tylenol over the counter. When he got back, her physician was amazed to find she had been manipulating him.

I had one young lady who had been a student off and on and was always trying to get pain drugs. I thought she was probably an addict, and I negotiated with her so that I would give her some Darvon every month without refills and she would check in each month. Eventually she turned up in the paper, dead from an overdose of heroin as is the fate of most addicts sooner or later.

One young woman whose family I knew socially called to ask if I would see her. She was a student but had insurance and had been seeing a private physician. She said she was having back trouble and was nearly incapacitated. Her physician had sent her to physical therapy and each time it seemed to make her hurt worse. I told her to come on in, and I'd do what I could. She arrived with her mother and told me this had been going on for three or four months. I knew this young woman was a horse woman and lived on a farm and was in good physical condition. When I asked where in her back she hurt, she pointed to her flank instead. Her back seemed normal, but even slight percussion on her flank caused excruciating pain. I examined her abdomen and found a mass a little smaller than a soccer ball on the side that was hurting. I sent her down for a stat ultrasound and found she had a huge cyst near her kidney. When I asked her, she admitted her physician had never actually examined her but just filled out the physical therapy referral. I referred her to a local urologist who was on her insurance panel, and he checked and found that kidney was still functioning. They took her to surgery and were able to repair what appeared to be a congenital stricture of her ureter on that side. All her pain went away.

One of the saddest things that occurred working with university faculty was watching them age. I had one patient who was retired but still very famous in his field whose wife came in in tears because he seemed to be losing his memory. I brought him in and talked with him, and although he was doing a good job of hiding it, he really was losing his memory. I referred him to a friend of mine who did testing for

Alzheimer's, and he confirmed this was the case. We put the patient on what medications there are and arranged for his wife to get some help in the home but could only tell her that he was probably going to get steadily worse. It's very hard to watch a great intellect just disappear before your eyes and be able to do very little to help. My own college professor father did the same thing.

A young Asian student came in one day complaining of a very sore throat. When I examined him I found he had exudate (pus) in his throat and a low-grade temp. As was standard I took a rapid strep test and told him how to manage his throat if the test wasn't positive. He returned the next day and saw another physician who told him his rapid strep test was negative and reaffirmed the instructions I'd given him the day before. When he returned the next day, he saw me again, and this time when I examined him, he had developed many cervical nodes, which are commonly found in infectious mononucleosis. I had hopes this would prove to be the case because we could start him on steroids, and the worst of his pain would be gone in a couple days. I sent him to the lab for a blood count and a mono test and told him I'd call him that afternoon. Later in the day I got a call from out chief lab tech to tell me he had eighty-six thousand white cells (top of normal is ten thousand) and they were mostly abnormal forms. She had sent the slide off for pathology review.

I called the young man and asked him to return to my office. Before he got there, the pathologist called to confirm that the slide looked like acute myeloginous leukemia. The last one of these I had seen was twenty years earlier and that patient had died in less than a week. When the patient got back to my office, I tried to explain to him what he had, but he really didn't have the vocabulary to totally understand. I finally got the concept of blood cancer through to him and told him he needed to go to the hospital right now. He asked if he could go to his dorm to get his laptop, and even though I told him time was very important, that's what he did. I had called my friend in Hematology-oncology and he'd had his fellow waiting to start treatment in the ER. As soon as the patient was available, he was on medication and was admitted. On the second day in the hospital the patient crashed and went into a coma and had to be put on a ventilator. If this had happened in his dorm room, he would have died, and he nearly died even in university hospital. He actually was given last rites three times before he came out of the coma. His family was scattered all over and had to fly in from China and Hong Kong, and his sister flew in from England where she was in grad school. The patient had bought student insurance, which had a half a million dollar limit. The hospital burned through that in the first week. Somehow they got him on Medicaid even though he was a foreign national. Once he woke up, they finished a full course of treatment and his bone marrow had gone back to normal. He left for home with completely normal labs but would have to be followed for years to be sure there was no recurrence. I was very glad he was persistent enough for us to pick up what was happening. I have to think of the thousands of sore throats seen in Health Service, and we were really lucky to pick up the one that wasn't mono or strep or a virus.

Because our students and faculty traveled all over the world, we had to be vigilant for the signs of the rare tropical diseases. Each year we'd have a case or two of malaria and we also found various worms. One young man was sent to me with a growth on his hand. He'd seen several physicians and none knew what he had. When I looked at it, I knew I'd never seen anything like it, and I decided to go ahead and do a small biopsy and see if the pathologist could help me. The patient told me the growth had started while he was in Bulgaria, but I could make nothing of that. Pathology called me to say the lesion was full of Leishmania, which is a parasite found in deserts and transmitted by the sand flea. This organism's primary host is a dog. When I called the patient back in, I found out that before going to Bulgaria, he had participated in an archeological dig in Jordan, which explained the source of the infestation. Fortunately for him he had the skin infestation rather than the fatal systemic form. Even so the only treatment was a drug you had to get from the CDC on a case-by-case basis. My friends in the Infectious Disease Department practically fought over the honor of treating this young man.

One day a lady came in who claimed to work for NASA. She told me she knew more than most of the engineers there but didn't have a degree so they wouldn't listen to her. She'd come to the university to get her degree so she could advance in her field. Naturally I was somewhat dubious about these claims but I saw no reason to challenge her. Since she felt she knew more than most of the professors, I suspected her time with us would not be a happy one. Over time she did end up in conflict with the professors as well as the administration, and I seemed to be the only person she would trust. I tried to send her for psychiatric help but she was unwilling to go. Eventually she was banned from campus, and all calls from her had to be referred to one of the lawyers in the Office of the university council. I always felt we'd failed to get her proper care, but with the lawyers involved there was little I could do.

By the time I reached sixty-five, I was ready to start slowing down. I officially retired from the university but was rehired as a "part-time temporary" and worked two more years half time before I totally stopped working.

Reflections

Over the forty odd years I've been in medicine the changes have been quite remarkable. The technology has changed dramatically for the better, but I think the compassion of the physicians has become less, and that's very sad. When I was in medical school, we had two diuretics and maybe three antihypertensive drugs. Today we have a large number of both available to us. We had x-ray but ultrasound, CT, MRI, and PET were all in the future. Digitalis was a common drug for heart failure and available in a number of forms. Today it is occasionally used for heart rhythm problems and only in one form. I haven't seen a case of digitalis toxicity in thirty years. We have pacemakers and implantable defibrillators. The cardiologist I externed with as a student still stopped (sometimes) atrial fibrillation by giving a drug until the fibrillation was controlled or the patient began uncontrolled vomiting. We expected a 5 percent rate of stillbirth when I started; whereas, today if you deliver a stillbirth, you have to go before a hospital committee and explain yourself. Caesarian Section was about 5 percent, but many, if not most, deliveries were with forceps (a technique many OB residents really have little or no training in today except a suction unit, a sort of plumber's friend for the infant's head). Modern C-section rates run close to 20 percent in some institutions.

We were taught that a 20 percent rate of negative appendectomies (appendectomies which found a normal appendix) was expected of a surgeon, and if he didn't have that rate, he was probably going to have some rupture. The surgery was always done open since we had no other way available. Now the use of ultrasound and helical CT has changed the whole diagnostic situation. We can actually see if the appendix is inflamed and swollen. Much modern surgery including appendectomy is done through scopes with minimal invasion.

The surgery that has had a most remarkable change is removing the gallbladder (cholecystectomy). The recovery time for this procedure done open was at least five days in the hospital followed by several weeks at home. Apparently most of the post-op problems were caused by the incision which involved cutting one of the rectus muscles. With the scope the muscles are intact and the patient is frequently out of the hospital in a day or two and back at work shortly thereafter.

In the office we had no computers when I started practice. When I formed the group, we were the first office in our area to computerize and that only for the business part of the practice. We put in an IBM 32 computer with the biggest memory they offered which, as I recall, was thirteen megabytes. We had to hire a programmer to write the program since there were no "off the shelf" programs for medical offices. We were able to sell that program to other offices to help make up the costs. Today the government has mandated all offices must be computerized not only for the business office but for the medical record as well. These programs suggest which drugs to use and which drugs will interact unfavorably. There are complicated algorithms such as if you enter that the patient has a cough there are suggested questions you should ask such as the presence of fever or spitting up blood. These do decrease the failure to reach the right diagnosis, and one wonders if doctors will be obsolete eventually.

I can't remember how many surgeries I assisted in to fix an ulcer and to cut the nerve to the stomach that seems to mediate acid release while also opening the exit from the stomach (called vagotomy and pyloroplasty) in an effort to prevent further ulcers. In fact when I was in the air force, a pilot could not return to flying after a bleeding ulcer unless this procedure was done. Today we know that almost all the stomach and duodenal ulcers are caused by a bacterium and can be cured using a combination of antibiotics.

One of the big differences in medicine is the change in therapeutics. A prime example is the difference in outcomes between the two patients I had with acute myologinous leukemia. The first lady lasted only four days from diagnosis and we were told her best case would be months of misery. The young man I diagnosed over twenty years later had either a cure or at least a complete remission. We are developing treatments for some viruses such as herpes zoster and more immunizations such as HPV. Unfortunately we're still in the situation that if the right virus comes along (Ebola, SARS, or Bird Flu), we could be right back in the middle ages with the only options being quarantine and burning houses. Most experts seem to feel that with modern transportation a pandemic is largely inevitable.

We have also become the victims of our own success with the advent of severely resistant strains of TB and Staph. We are therefore in an arms race with the microbes of the world, and the old-fashioned treatments of draining abscesses, isolation, hand washing and control of fomites (contaminated bedding, clothing etc.) has developed renewed importance. We have numerous organisms in our hospitals that are harder and harder to treat, and we must use great care to avoid what I witnessed in Guatemala where you didn't die from what you were hospitalized for but rather from what you caught in the hospital.

Since we had to get rid of DDT we now have bed bugs back. When the first case of these nasty things came into the Health Service, I was the only physician old enough to remember the bite pattern. Since that time they have spread rapidly and most primary care clinicians should recognize them.

We can now replace hips, knees, ankles, and shoulders as well as transplant hearts, lungs, kidneys, livers, corneas, and even whole faces. We are implanting devices to replace hearing and vision and are making great progress in being able to regrow many different tissues. Cataract surgery has become simple and commonplace. We have gone from total mastectomy (breast removal) to simple mastectomy with replacement and frequently only require lumpectomy.

Prosthetics have taken a quantum jump in particular because of the Iraq war. We have also defined what PTSD is and have begun to recognize minimal brain damage. We have numerous treatments for clinical depression, a disorder which had a 25 percent death rate from suicide in the past.

Obstetrics has gone both ways with more nurse midwives and home births to constant fetal monitoring and fetal scalp pH sampling. We have birthing rooms with cosmetic frilly bed covers with thousands of dollars of high-tech equipment hidden in bedside tables. Our C-section rates have been climbing and it's almost become an alternative delivery method. We keep mothers in the hospital two or three days and we recently had to fight off insurance companies who wanted "drive-through" deliveries. When I was an intern, we required a fourteen-day stay. That stay was a self-fulfilling prophecy in that being in bed that long produced the leg clots we were watching for.

The result of all these changes seems to me to have been a tendency, especially in some specialties, for the residents to become more scientific and less compassionate. I think this may have something to do with the training they receive since my students don't seem to show this tendency as much. Many, if not most, of the professors in medical school are research oriented and consider patient care to be secondary. I've been told by some of the best clinicians in the university that they've been threatened because they don't spend enough time doing research. When a professor spends half a day a week doing clinic and the rest of his time doing research, he has a bias toward research. There is absolutely no correlation between good research and good teaching either. I would like to see the medical schools split their faculty between clinical and research and then pick the best teachers from both groups. They should also spend some more time in medical ethics and doctor-patient relationships.

The Hippocratic Oath was developed from a philosophy expounded by a number of ancient Greek physicians, one of whom was probably named Hippocrates. The philosophy was patient oriented and holds to this day but is seldom mentioned in modern medical schools. The idea that holding a patient's hand or just sitting and talking with them is as important therapeutically as fancy drugs and tests just doesn't seem to come up. When I try with my few students to encourage this, they seem very responsive to the idea, and I hope they become better clinicians because of it. This does not mean they should ignore science and give the patient everything they want whether it is good for them or not. I see far too many physicians who freely give antibiotics when they are not indicated just because the patient believes they will help.

This is the easy way out rather than trying to educate the patient that this is not good for him or society in general. I suspect the extreme version of this becomes the doctors who prescribe narcotics and other meds excessively. These physicians missed the expression of "first do no harm." It is certainly easier to write a prescription than take the time to discuss with the patient why this is a bad idea. I've heard physicians say if they didn't do it, the patient would find someone who would. I think this expresses a very poor self-image that you must do something you know is wrong because if you don't someone else will. I think sometimes it's also the worry that the patient will move on, and you will lose the billings. Some of the most extreme of these cases include Elvis and Michael Jackson, but you have to wonder how many non-famous people die from medications that were prescribed inappropriately and were simply covered up by the docs themselves on the death certificates.

We continue to fight the battle of ever increasing medical costs. Our culture has become yet another leg in what used to be a three legged stool. We are battling an epidemic of obesity from too much food and not enough exercise. The result is a huge increase in the complications of obesity including diabetes and hypertension. Obesity has always been a very difficult problem to treat and isn't getting easier. Any time you try to change people's lifestyle, you meet incredible resistance. The people we have elected think they can do better, and I wish them good luck but would be astounded if they are successful.

Another contributor to health care costs is malpractice. At one point in my career I was paying around $60,000 a year for my malpractice insurance and wasn't taking home much more than that. Many frivolous suits are filed to try to get the insurance company to settle. If the company can settle for $100,000, they will save money over going to trial, and the lawyer filing the suit will get $30,000 or more. There's no disincentive for him to try except the minor costs of filing.

When I was starting out it was a breach of ethics for a lawyer to advertise. Today the airways are full of ads for law firms who will sue if anything doesn't work perfectly. The criteria are no longer malpractice but mal-result. If the physician does everything right and the patient has a side effect or doesn't heal right, the physician will be sued. We actually had a patient file her own suit against one of my partners because her posterior hurt after delivering a large healthy baby. Lawsuits look like easy money to a small part of the population and a larger part of the legal community.

The ultimate solution to health care costs is going to be a very bitter pill. Short of rationing care we will probably never be able to control costs. I once had an insurance company executive tell me that you can't get a Cadillac by paying for a Chevrolet, and yet Americans all expect Cadillac medicine at all times for themselves and for their relatives. Even when elderly patients decide they've had enough, their families can be insistent on doing everything possible, and doctors and hospitals are so afraid of lawsuits they are reluctant to pull the plug if even one relative objects. The reasons for the refusal of relatives to allow loved ones to go are sometimes startling. I heard one ethicist tell about a man who was on breathing machines and all kinds of support. The family had all agreed not to prolong the situation since there was no hope of any recovery. The only person who objected was his wife. When the ethicist explained to the wife that keeping this man on life support was just prolonging his suffering, she said, "Wal, I don't reckon he's suffered near enough yet." Family dynamics can be very different from what you'd suppose.

On a personal note, while I was doing all these things we were also raising six children and I think they came out very well probably more the result of my wife's influence than their chronically absent father's. At the time this is being written they have all left home and are doing well.

Doug, our oldest, is a career NCO in the army and is deploying to Afghanistan again. This is his fourth overseas assignment. By the third his marriage broke up, as is so common among our military, but he's progressing in his career. Doug has two children, a girl and a boy who live across the country, and we have only minimal contact with them, which we find very frustrating.

Thanh, our oldest girl, graduated in food science and was a field investigator for many years with the FDA. After she married, her husband had to go to Naples, Italy, and she gave up her job but now she's finishing her Master's degree in Human Relations and is looking for employment in that field either in Italy or back in the United States.

Vinh, our younger boy, had polio in Vietnam and came over essentially paralyzed from the waist down. He became an alcoholic and crack addict but he had the strength to get himself clean years ago and the family is very proud of him. Unfortunately he now is battling chronic depression and post-polio syndrome, which can cause a problem with pain and poor co-ordination. He is, however, able to live on his own and still is working toward his goal of becoming a drug and alcohol counselor.

Bridget graduated from college with a degree in political science and went to work in Al Gore's vice-presidential office answering correspondence. She subsequently got a job working for Congressman David Bonier when he was House minority whip. After he retired, she went back to law school and now works as a lawyer for Legal Aid where she specializes in representing children with mental disabilities. She has two delightful little boys and her husband works as the CEO of a small think-tank.

Erin was born a congenital triple amputee with only one arm. In spite of that she became a horse woman in high school and participated in the state equestrian championship team for all four years she was in high school. She went on to get her degree in psychology and then went to Ohio and got a PsyD. She then did a fellowship in rehab psychology and currently works for the VA as a rehabilitation psychologist. She is still part owner in an Arabian horse. She has just recently presented us with our fifth grandchild.

Kathleen graduated from college in violin performance and is currently working on a master's degree in music as well as getting certified in Suzuki violin.

I suppose I should say something about my thoughts about the future of medicine. I have no crystal ball but some trends seem predictable. I see medicine sadly becoming more and more impersonal. Your physician no longer cares for you in the hospital but turns your care over to a hospitalist who knows nothing about you. This person doesn't follow-up after you leave so really doesn't know if the care was appropriate or not. In the systems I'm familiar with, there seems to be very little communication between the primary physician and the hospitalist even though the information is often on a computer system accessible to both. Perhaps we need to require the primary physician to approve the reports within a specified time.

Computers can take a history and make a diagnosis more accurately than a trained internist. The MRI coupled with a diagnostic program may be more accurate than a physical exam.

We will soon be able to make changes in human genetic code and therefore eliminate tendencies for cancer and other diseases as well as correct various single-gene disorders.

We will be able to grow new parts such as skin, bone, tendons, and many others as well as whole organs from the patient's own stem cells thereby avoiding the whole problem of tissue rejection in transplants.

I suspect the field of nanotechnology will play a large role in the future as well as other new technologies with which I'm not even familiar.

Unfortunately this will all cost money and keep people living longer thus increasing medical costs until we will be unable to offer everything to everyone and we will almost certainly have to resort to more overt rationing than we have not.

We can only hope there will be a breakthrough in costs as well because the future of the science of medicine is rosy indeed.

www.ingramcontent.com/pod-product-compliance
Lightning Source LLC
Chambersburg PA
CBHW020734180526
45163CB00001B/227
* 9 7 8 1 4 9 9 0 1 5 4 0 9 *